THRIVING! is the only book of its kind! It is a remarkable combination of stories from surgical weight loss patients and a thorough education about biological and psychological aspects of obesity. *THRIVING!* is a must-read for anyone considering weight loss surgery, for those who have had surgery, and for anyone struggling with obesity. This is a book of compassion about those who suffer from the deadly disease of obesity.

Garth Davis, MD
Bariatric Surgeon
The Davis Clinic, Houston, TX

"If you are going through a struggle with weight, whether or not you have chosen bariatric surgery as your weight-loss tool, this book is a must-read. Dr. Stapleton approaches the issues with both compassion and clarity and has compiled amazing stories from people who are fighters and are finding solutions to obesity that work for life. Connie is so good at digging deep and understanding the underlying causes of obesity. She focuses on treating the deeper issues. Working with her is always such a pleasure and an honor. My clients love her work and can feel her passion for helping others. This book is another great example of just that!"

Erin Akey, CPT, WFI, FNC
"The Bariatric Guru"
Host, "Fit Living" radio

"Dr. Connie Stapleton is the only person who could pull off this kind of book. Why? She "gets" us! She is not just an advocate for us, she cares and becomes a genuine friend. You will not find a better person to have not only in your corner, but also at your side helping you on your journey back to health—physically and mentally."

z
t

D1218235

"I wish this book had been available when I was morbidly obese because my doctor *might* have told me to move more, eat less AND . . . *go to therapy.*

In my opinion, *THRIVING!* should be mandatory reading for anyone who thinks losing weight is a matter of character."

Cari De La Cruz
Blogger, Speaker and Gastric Bypass Post-Op (2007)

"This is a book that had to be written. It is a great encouragement as well as a challenge to everyone who wears the battle scar of obesity. It is a book of hope as patients share their hearts. Dr. Stapleton was the best one to write it—she knows the heart of the morbidly obese."

Laura Van Tuyl
CEO Living Healthy For a Lifetime

"It took years to find a professional that "gets us" and was willing to work in the trenches with those of us who knew how much more there was to know about our disease. Dr. Connie Stapleton was willing to listen to us, sort out our street credential knowledge and help patients and pros communicate better so we could trust each other and learn how important our heads are in this journey. It begins and ends with our brain and Connie explains it in our own words!"

Yvonne McCarthy
BariatricGirl.com,
Volunteer Heath and Wellness Coach,
Speaker, Gastric Bypass (2001)

THRIVING!

TRIUMPH *over* TRAUMA

REAL LIFE STORIES OF RECOVERY FROM OBESITY

CONNIE
STAPLETON, PhD

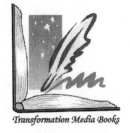

Transformation Media Books

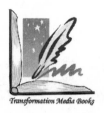

Transformation Media Books

Published by Transformation Media Books, USA
www.TransformationMediaBooks.com

An imprint of Pen & Publish, Inc.
Bloomington, Indiana
(812) 837-9226
info@PenandPublish.com
www.PenandPublish.com

Cover design by Cari De La Cruz
Text design by Jane Hagaman

ISBN: 978-0-9852737-8-1

This book is printed on acid free paper.

Printed in the United States

DEDICATION

For every person who has known the pain, be it physical, emotional, or both, associated with obesity, find peace in these words. And then live them:

"Life is an opportunity; benefit from it.
Life is beauty; admire it.
Life is a dream; realize it.
Life is a challenge; meet it.
Life is a duty; complete it.
Life is a game; play it.
Life is a promise; fulfill it.
Life is sorrow; overcome it.
Life is a song; sing it.
Life is a struggle; accept it.
Life is a tragedy; confront it.
Life is an adventure; dare it.
Life is luck; make it.
Life is too precious; do not destroy it.
Life is life; fight for it."

Mother Teresa

"Yesterday is gone. Tomorrow has not yet come. We have only today. Let us begin."

Mother Teresa

ACKNOWLEDGMENTS

This book would not have come to fruition without Antonia Namnath, founder and CEO of the Weight Loss Surgery Foundation of America (WLSFA), so my personal thanks go to Antonia. Not just for her enthusiasm, support, and help in getting the stories for this book, but for her inspiration, bravery, and determination to spearhead the WLSFA. Toni—you are a remarkable woman whom I admire and respect. Thanks for all you do to help so many.

Rosemary Almgren and Connie Bailey—you two are the actual inspiration for this book! When I watched the WLSFA documentary about the two of you, my imagination was immediately sparked. The courage you demonstrated by sharing the personal, painful truth related to your obesity was powerful. I instantly knew that your willingness to talk about the abusive past you survived would help inform hundreds of others about the psychological connection between emotional pain and obesity. I was completely impressed by the two of you. Now that I know you, I am even more impressed, as you are both sincere, down-to-earth, playful, loving women who are heroes. "Thank you" seems like two very small words when I think of the impact you have had on the lives of so many. My personal gratitude to you both for inspiring this book, and for being willing to contribute to it, is heartfelt. Many thanks for the ongoing help you give to other obese people who need hope and to the hundreds of formerly obese people you continue to encourage on their journey. You set a phenomenal example to us all on how to live life fully and to love unconditionally.

To every person who contributed their stories, their creative work, their blog posts, and parts of themselves—this book is truly the result of your contributions. Thank you for being so generous as to share your intensely personal journeys so others may have the courage to follow in your footsteps. Thank you for taking your own steps toward better health. Thank you for allowing me into your lives; I consider it a privilege to be privy to your worlds. Thank you for trusting your peers to read about your journeys; may they glean hope and the courage to travel outside their comfort zones to find a greater level of health and peace. Thank you, too, for leading your families and loved ones to healthier lives—in all aspects of their worlds. To the clients who allowed me to print your "home-work" in this book—I thank you for trusting me and for working through very important issues with me. You are very special to me.

A very special thank you to the great friends I have made in my work with the WLS community. I appreciate you helping me out in so many ways, and in this case, for graciously agreeing to open your private worlds up to the public by sharing your stories and your writings with everyone. Cari, you are my business buddy and a trusted friend. The book cover, which you personally envisioned and designed, is a mere sample of your brilliance—not only with words but all things creative. "Thank you" does not begin to express my gratitude for your contribution to the WLS community and especially for being my business partner! My work is truly only half as good without you! Erin—you are the other person with whom I collaborate and are also a new, true friend. Yvonne—you are one of the best people I have ever known; I genuinely believe you are an angel put on this earth. Carla—you are a mighty example of a leader in the WLS community, and I have learned much from you; thank you for always encouraging me and so often leading the way!

Very special thank-yous to my husband, Steve, and daughter, Kelsey, who read and reread and then read the manuscript some more. I appreciate your patience, your keen eyes, which caught so many of my mistakes, and your great suggestions. To my son, Steven, and my daughter, Erin, and all of my family and my bestest friends, thank you for loving me and continuing to support all of my endeavors. Most especially, thank you for sharing our lives and our families. A very biased thank you to my brand new grandson, Gummy Bear, for making me wear a smile in my heart every day for the three months since you were born (and to your parents for generously sharing your life with us!).

To everyone reading this book, thank you for your time. Thank you for sharing this with others! And thank you for taking into consideration the information in this book that "fits" for you. May it inform you, encourage you, and inspire you to make your own life healthier in every way!

TABLE OF CONTENTS

FOREWORD

I met Dr. Connie Stapleton the way a lot of weight loss surgery patients do, at an obesity event. She was there as a speaker and also hosted a table where she greeted the many fans of her book, *Eat It Up!* Like all the others in line, I was so excited to meet Dr. Stapleton and have her sign my copy of her book. I had no idea that day we would become true friends and that one day she would author a book that would actually benefit the Weight Loss Surgery Foundation of America—WLSFA.

As the founder of the WLSFA, I have crisscrossed the country, attending obesity events to spread the word about our beloved charity. Connie is always there too, educating and motivating people. Always with a warm smile and kind heart, she listens as people pour their hearts out. I admire Connie more than she could ever know. Her poise and grace make her shine even in a crowded convention center.

When Connie proposed writing a book that would gather the real stories and voices of morbid obesity and weight loss surgery patients, I was already thrilled. Educating people about morbid obesity is one of the core missions of the WLSFA. When Connie said she would contribute a huge portion of the profits to the WLSFA, I was beside myself with joy.

I am so happy the book is now published and am overjoyed you

are reading this because it means you will understand OUR COM-
MUNITY better. You will read stories that will touch your heart and
make you understand just how complex obesity is. This book will
do more to confront the negative bias against people who suffer
from obesity than any other book on the market because this book
is REALITY TV in book form. It is our real experience, pain, and
triumph over the monster that is the disease of obesity.

If you are a fellow WLS Peep, thank you for purchasing this
book. It helps the WLSFA accomplish our core mission to fund
grants for weight loss and reconstructive surgery! Together we are
saving lives one grant at a time! If you are a person suffering from
obesity and looking for solutions to take your life and health back,
I urge you to read this book and share it with your loved ones.
Know you are NOT ALONE and that we, the weight loss patient
community, are here to help you learn, are here for you to lean
on, and will cheer you on no matter what path you take to health!

—Antonia Namnath
CEO and Founder
Weight Loss Surgery Foundation of America
WLSFA.ORG

CHAPTER ONE

"My name is Rosemary Almgren, and this is my weight loss surgery story.

My twin sister, Connie, and I started our lives on the third day of March, 1962. Our parents were both of Mexican descent. Our father was from Guadalajara, Mexico, and [our] mother was from Grulla, Texas. They both wanted a better life for themselves and for their children, so they uprooted and came to Dallas, Texas, where they had seven children. Five boys and my sister and me.

Life was hard for my parents because my father was a lawyer in Mexico, and my mother was going to nursing school in her hometown. My father found a job with a growing company as a factory worker. Life was hard, but good. Mother was a great cook and used traditional cooking methods from her past, which included lots of fats and carbs. Flour or corn tortillas [were] our bread of the day, and bread was part of every meal.

As we grew, I noticed my brothers were thin, and yet my sister and I were fat. I remember as a child asking God, 'Why?' And I remember wanting foods like the other children in our neighborhood had. They ate hot dogs and hamburgers. We never ate those things unless we were invited to someone else's home, where they just happened to give us a quick bite to eat.

Then tragedy struck our lives. My father died in 1967. My sister and I were only four-and-a-half years old. This made things only get rougher for our family. My brothers were still thin, and [we] girls were only getting fatter. The boys were all forced to find work to help out with our family bills. Some got married at a young age and left home. We grew up eating a lot of unhealthy items. And life went on.

Mother found herself lonely and would venture out with different men who were invited to stay in our home at times. This was never a good idea because they tried many times to touch me. This resulted in my eating more, which caused my weight to balloon. My sister and I never talked about what was happening to us as children. When we grew up, we found out that the same things happened to one another. We were both in terrible pain at the same time but never found the courage to speak of it.

We went on to finish high school. Life was beginning for both of us. Connie was married after high school at the age of 18. I was married at the age of 19. It seems that marrying at a young age is a pattern in our family. Connie was pregnant the first year of her marriage. Her weight began to balloon as she ate things like stuffing, which she could not get enough of. Her weight became more and more of an issue as she grew even heavier. I'm not sure, but this might have contributed to her delivering a large child, who weighed 11 pounds at birth. Her second child weighed 10.8 pounds.

Connie maintained the same poor eating habits with food throughout her second pregnancy. Connie and I were pregnant at the same time for two months. Our children are seven months apart. She had two girls, and I had two girls.

Not only did we grow up eating unhealthily, but now we were adults ourselves and had begun cooking unhealthy meals for our own families. Both of our husbands were used to authentic Mexican food. Connie's relationship with her first husband was very rocky and unstable. This resulted in continued unhealthy eating, and the pounds kept packing on.

My relationship with my husband was even worse. I had very low self-esteem, and was told many times by my husband that if I was not so lazy that I could lose weight. Those comments only caused more pain and resulted in more pounds. Our lives were so unhappy, and the future held even more rough patches that yes, resulted in even more weight gain for both of us.

Connie was divorced in 1989, and she started to regain her smile and strength. She found some success with a diet and lost enough weight to feel good about herself. She then met her knight in shining armor. He not only took on her children, but our mother as well. Connie had lots of pressures with a new marriage and family. At the same time, yet again tragedy struck, as our mother was diagnosed with breast cancer. This made matters worse.

As the stress of life became too much for her, Connie again found herself failing to maintain a good weight. The pounds began to slowly creep right back on, year after year. Three years before my mother passed away, she came to live with me. I was already much heavier then Connie, and I also found myself drowning in food as I tried to relieve the stress of everyday life.

Then life came crashing down! My mother lost her battle with cancer in March of 1998. I was alone, and my emotions were out of control when my husband told me that he was in love with another woman. But he would not give me a divorce. I felt trapped and lost. Again, food was my only friend and comforter. I had ballooned to 447 pounds.

One day when I was working at the school, I fell and was not able to get up by my own means. It was very painful, embarrassing, and humiliating to see that some of my students stood and watched as it took four men, along with my daughter, to pick me up. This was my breaking point. I said I had to do something. Anything was better than how I was living because this was not living. I was only existing.

So in May of 1999, I began my weight loss journey with the Atkins diet. I studied the book and did everything I could to stay on track. I found that I was being successful for the first time and was losing weight at a great pace. In August of 1999, only three months into refocusing and changing the way I was eating, my husband died of a heart attack. I was left alone with two children to raise.

It seemed as if life was always full of ups and downs and curves. But this time I said I would not fail. I looked to God for strength and to keep me focused enough to not have the death of my husband keep me from succeeding. It was hard, and many people said to me that it was impossible to not regain my weight. But I had to prove them wrong. I had to do this for me this time.

I was starting to love the woman I was becoming, inside and out. During the first year I lost 100 pounds, and not one person noticed. I still had a long way to go, but I was determined it would happen. The second year, I lost another 100 pounds. I was now 247 pounds. I started to get noticed by men and worked even harder. I dated some, but did not like the fact that at the end of a date they wanted so much more. I was not going to go there. One day I passed a glass window and saw my reflection. I could not believe what I was seeing looking back at me! Why did I not do this sooner?! It was hard to see my smaller reflection. But I promised myself that I would never go back to being so heavy and unhappy.

Later, in December of 2002, I met my blue-eyed Eric. We met in a Christian chat room. I was scared because of the men I had dated before, so we took it slowly and only talked by Internet or phone. I weighed 172 pounds then. We decided to meet for the first time face-to-face on February 14, Valentine's Day. It was a fast courtship. He asked me to marry him in March, and I began starving myself to get down to 147 pounds, which I did reach on my wedding day. I saw that weight for about a week! On my honeymoon, I started to pack the pounds on again. It was like there was no control. I said, 'Well, I'll start the Atkins program again when I return to Dallas.' But it was already spiraling out of control. I regained up to 265 pounds. Eric knew I was beside myself and was feeling like I had no hope. He sent me to his doctor, who heard my story of weight loss and regain.

The doctor thought I should go see a friend of hers who is a gastric bypass surgeon. At the same time, Connie was also looking into gastric bypass, but I had no idea. I was approved for surgery within two weeks, but she was denied. When we spoke about this, we were both in shock that we had worked on having the exact same procedure done. I was given the chance to change my life for the better, and she was sadly denied. Her life would remain the same. While my life moved on and my body began to shrink again after surgery, I was positive that she would get approval soon. She tried other policies and was denied again and again. She was denied a total of three times. It was as if I was on a moving sidewalk and she was on a regular sidewalk, trying to catch up with the use of her own strength and willpower. But she was not getting anywhere. Her efforts with the insurance companies were all in vain, for each time she was given hope, but to no avail. It was very hard for me to see my life go on with change for the better and to watch hers stay the same. I so wanted to see her change as I did."

Your Peers Tell the Real Story

The moment I finished watching the documentary *Surviving to Thriving,* presented by the Weight Loss Surgery Foundation of

America (WLSFA), featuring Rosemary Almgren (whose story you read above) and her twin sister, Connie Bailey, I called Antonia Namnath, founder and CEO of WLSFA. "Toni," I began, excitedly, "I am beyond amazed at Rosemary's and Connie's story! These women are so incredibly brave and inspirational! They are talking about the underlying issues related to their obesity. To begin with, their father passed away when they were only four years old. They were just babies! They talk about the food-related memories they have of their father. Even at that early age, they were developing an emotional relationship with food. Dad brought crackers for them, which they associated with love and their father's returning home from work each day. Even more courageously, they spoke openly in the documentary about having been sexually abused by men their mother brought into the house as she was "trying to find a Dad for us," Rosemary reported. Connie added, "The men my mother would bring into the home. . . . She thought they were these nice men. And, um . . . they weren't." In the video Toni boldly prints, *"Like so many who suffer from obesity, Rosemary and Connie were victims of sexual trauma."*

Rosemary spoke of seeing the tremendous pain her mother was in and didn't want to burden her further by telling her about the men who were abusing Connie and her. She noted that the abuse occurred "more than once" and stated, "I think that's when food began to comfort me. That's when I would run and hide because this was all done in secret. So food was done in secret. That's when I took food and would comfort myself. And that's how I took care of the situation. What I was doing was . . . I was creating a bigger body. A bigger shell. A bigger shell. A bigger shell. And that's how I reached 447 pounds."

I continued on my phone call with Toni, rambling on with enthusiasm I could barely contain. "Oh my goodness, Toni—these women are so, so, so brave to share this information! And thank you and the WLSFA and Bariatric TV for making public what so many people feel the need to keep private. These two women are giving people such a gift. Actually, many gifts! The gift to acknowledge and talk about the pain of being abused. And the gift of enabling others to make the connection of having used food to deal with painful emotions. In Rosemary's and Connie's cases, food was used to deal with painful emotions and to build a body in which to escape being abused by other men. Toni, this message, coming from these beautiful women, may give others the courage to discover the relationship between obesity and emotional pain, to face their pain, to deal with it, and therefore heal from it."

Then I asked Toni the question that had led me to pick up the phone and call her, "How about if we ask others to share their stories about what contributed to their obesity, and then write a book using their information? Money from the book will go to the WLSFA so that others, like Connie, who can't afford to pay for weight loss surgery on their own and who don't have insurance that covers WLS, can have it via the WLSFA. Hopefully, we can help others find the courage to acknowledge any emotional pain they have related to their obesity, dredge up the courage to address their pain, and consequently, heal from it and make keeping the weight off after surgery much easier!" (Okay, say maybe I didn't say all that in exactly those words, but that was the gist of what I was thinking—and trying to say!) Without hesitation, Toni agreed to help get the word out to gather stories for the book.

I put together a short form with some questions to help people think about their lives, their obesity, and how their lives have changed since having weight loss surgery. What I got was so much more than I could have asked for! People shared their hearts, their lives, their pain, their secrets, their struggles, their victories, and their joys. Like Rosemary and Connie, these incredible people, both men and women, all shared their experiences in the hope of helping others. All I can say about that is, "How truly amazing *is* that?"

In this book, you will hear some of the worst about humanity, but will also witness through words, the remarkable strength, resilience, and goodness of humanity. You will feel the generosity of each of these people who revealed their experiences, how they dealt with adversity and bravely opted to make positive changes in their lives and the lives of their families when they chose to have weight loss surgery. Feel and share the hope they offer and pass it on, as they have done by contributing to this book. Read in here the best about humanity.

It is important for me to make sure you know that I have not changed or altered the information provided by the contributors, other than to make minor editorial changes. Their messages are intact. I was astounded as I read the submissions I received from people. I thought, "This is by far the best way to write a book! It's one thing for a psychologist to talk about this or that. But when the people who have walked the walk do the talking, it is so much more powerful than anything I could ever say! It's so true. Your peers tell the *real* story!" I thank each of you from the bottom of my heart. You will reach people who might not otherwise hear the messages in this book. Thank you. Thank you.

Due to the incredibly personal nature of the information in these stories, even though many of the participants were willing to use their real names, I have chosen to make all but a few of the contributors anonymous. You will understand why as you read further.

I am certain you will share my gratitude for the generous contributions of each of the "authors" of this book. I am privileged to be the person compiling and organizing their stories into a few chapters that will hopefully increase your knowledge about obesity, inspire you to delve into any issues you have related to your obesity, lead you to whatever additional help you need to heal from past hurts, and motivate you to share your insights and wisdom with others who are on the journey of recovering from obesity. If you know people who are currently struggling with obesity, encourage them to read this book. They will feel less isolated knowing that many others have had thoughts, feelings, and experiences similar to theirs and have been down many of the same roads they are presently treading. Perhaps they, too, will consider having weight loss surgery and open their lives to unlimited possibilities.

In addition to wanting to share the stories of those who opted to contribute to this book, I want it to be a learning tool. For those readers who have already had weight loss surgery, my hope is that you will give yourself permission to acknowledge any pain you have carried which resonates with the experiences shared by others who have figuratively walked in your shoes. Take the opportunity to talk to a friend, a religious leader, or a professional therapist if you need to. Working through your issues frees you of carrying them with you. In addition, it helps soothe the intensity of what sometimes feels like an "urgent need" to eat, which may, in reality, be your body's way of saying, "Pay attention! I am your buried feelings, and I need you to tend to me!" Eating sometimes represents an attempt to stuff the painful feelings down—again.

If you are overweight or obese but have not had weight loss surgery, my hope is that you, too, will read the experiences of those who contributed to this book with an open heart. Whether or not you ever have weight loss surgery, you have the opportunity to rid yourself of painful emotions that may be related to your weight issues. Doing so may make your weight loss endeavors more successful as you will no longer need to "eat at" unpleasant memories and feelings. Read with an open mind the information I provide which the contributors have shared through their personal stories. Apply what fits to your life to help make your weight loss efforts more successful.

If you do not, or have not ever had a weight problem and are reading this book, please read with compassion. Recognize the pain that obese people suffer when people stare, make critical comments, and judge them unfairly. Encourage others to treat this group of human beings with the same amount of respect every person deserves. Learn about the disease of morbid obesity, separating fact from fiction. Please help educate others so we can work as a unified community in our efforts to prevent and reduce obesity.

The following blog post by a well-known blogger in the WLS world, Cari De La Cruz, was written without any connection to the documentary featuring Rosemary and Connie, but it's also about the idea of surviving or thriving in relation to weight:

Surviving, Striving or Thriving— Thriving in the Bariatric After Life

When I chose to have gastric bypass surgery, I didn't realize what a radical, utter and permanent effect it would have on my life. As I settled into a new way of thinking, eating and being, I took on the attitude of a survivor; one who clung to life by her very fingertips, only relinquishing the death grip long enough to take the next authorized sip of water or small bite of food.

But I took it all in stride, never complaining about my decision to have weight loss surgery, or lamenting the strange circumstances in which I now found myself. It was an oddly surreal existence—or more aptly SUBsistence. I had become a person who spent each day just trying to survive from one hour to the next. It's true, this new life of survival paid handsome dividends on the scale, in my closet, and in my life. But, I was so focused on surviving, it never occurred to me that I should seek something greater. That is not to say that I didn't have profound and long-lasting satisfaction in my life—because I did. It's just that I was no longer looking for happiness in the food I was consuming, as all too often, when I ate something I thought would bring pleasure, all I got was pain. And I wasn't expecting to enjoy my active life, because so many things had transpired to set me back (injuries, surgeries, etc.), I figured it would always be a literal and figurative uphill climb; a slog.

Essentially, I spent my first year after surgery STRIVING to SURVIVE. I was striving NOT to throw up, striving to get enough protein in, striving to drink enough fluid each day, striving to remain active, striving to find clothes that would fit, striving to correct people who believed I'd taken the "easy way out," striving to find balance in a crazy new life.

But something happened in year two: The strive to survive had been replaced by the desire to THRIVE.

Somewhere along the way, I began to see life through a whole new paradigm.

The "before" Cari would fall off the horse and never get back on. I would starve my way through a diet plan until I couldn't take the deprivation another day, then I'd "eat something bad," and throw the towel in on the whole thing. Or, I'd start an exercise program, but I'd miss one day, which would quickly turn into two days, three days . . . a week, until it was "too late" to go back.

Why should I hope for success when I'd lived nothing but "failure" for my whole life? But looking at it now, I realized that I had a pattern of failure because I was willing to give up too easily. Never mind the fact that the failure was self-imposed, that I was sabotaging myself at every turn, or that I errantly believed I was entitled to success. All I knew was, exercise didn't work, diets were torture, and behavior modification was for the "results not typical" crowd.

But surgery threw open the doors to an entirely new way of thinking, and the "after" Cari quickly learned that physical discipline takes constant effort, but pays off.

At the end of the day, making healthy food choices, planning my meals, getting regular exercise and attending weekly support group meetings really has effected a radical and transformative change in my life. Dare I say, I've learned to THRIVE, and not just SURVIVE?

- Where are you in your weight loss journey?
- Are you still laboring to survive by keeping your nose to the diet and exercise grindstone, or have you found a way to thrive through healthy eating and an active lifestyle?
- Have you integrated a new way thinking into your new, fit self, or are you still thinking and acting like an unhealthy obese person?
- Are you barely SURVIVING in life?
- Are you STRIVING to lead a healthier and happier life?
- Have you learned to THRIVE in your new after life?

Surviving is something you do because you HAVE to.
Striving is something you do because you CHOOSE to.
Thriving is something you do because you WANT to.

Are you a SURVIVOR, a STRIVER, or a THRIVER?

—Blog post by Cari De La Cruz
(www.bariatricafterlife.com)

Obesity hurts. Recovering from obesity heals—physically, emotionally, and spiritually. Near the end of the documentary *Surviving to Thriving*, Rosemary says to Connie, "You're going to get a chance to be the most awesome person. The healthy person that you want to be. And you're going to be able to live the life that you've always wanted. And we're going to live together." She goes on to say, through joyful tears, "We're going to be able to walk together. Side by side. . . . We're going to get on a plane together and go somewhere. That's what I want. I want you to experience what I'm experiencing."

Read on to learn about the remarkable experiences of other post-ops, both prior to and after making the healthy decision to have weight loss surgery.

CHAPTER TWO

Believe me when I tell you that weight loss surgery
is NOT the easy way out!

In fact, it's the opposite.

This is not something you do for a year and then quit.
This is for life!

Weight Loss Surgery—the "Easy Way"

I have heard this sentiment, wisely stated in the quote above by one of the contributors to this book, and hundreds of times from surgical weight loss patients. It's interesting how many people admit to me during their pre-surgical psychological evaluation, that prior to seriously considering surgery they, too, said, "Weight loss surgery is the easy way out." As post-ops, they know the reality—there is nothing easy about going through the process of weight loss surgery and living the "bariatric after life," as my good friend, business partner (in A Post Op & A Doc), and successful post-op, Cari De La Cruz, calls life after weight loss surgery (www.bariatricafterlife. com). Sadly, there *are* scores of people who do believe that weight loss surgery is "*the easy way.*"

I have yet to hear even one post-op tell me, "Yep! By golly—this weight loss surgery process *is* the easy way, for sure!" Post-ops know the incredible time, effort, and hard work they have put into the pre-surgical process. More importantly, they are acutely aware of the difficulties associated with the post-op process. It's frequently far more difficult dealing with "life issues" following surgery than any biological problems related to the surgery itself! The decision to have weight loss surgery. . . . The process of preparing for weight loss surgery. . . . The lifelong process of keeping the weight off after surgery. . . . Dealing with the emotional issues related to losing a lot of weight in a relatively short amount of time. . . . Easy? Not a chance.

Here are a few analogies to consider:

- Is a cigarette smoker who takes Chantix or Wellbutrin or uses a nicotine patch to end the self-destruction caused by cigarettes *taking the easy way out?*

- Is an alcoholic who goes through an inpatient or outpatient treatment program to stop drinking *taking the easy way out?*

- Is a prescription or illegal drug addict who seeks medical assistance and a treatment program to stop using drugs *taking the easy way out?*

- Is a compulsive shopper whose spending has led to financial distress *taking the easy way out* by utilizing the services of a financial management company?

- Is a couple having marital difficulties *taking the easy way out* by seeking professional counseling?

I think the consensus would be that the people described above would be doing a great thing for themselves (and their loved ones) by *getting help* to quit smoking, by *getting medical and emotional support* to stop drinking or using other drugs, by *seeking assistance* to learn how to manage finances, or by *securing help* from a professional to learn healthy communication skills and other tools to enjoy a healthy marriage. In fact, I would venture to say that friends and family members would tell these people, "I'm proud of you for getting the help that you need." (Oh, and if your loved ones don't express enthusiasm regarding your efforts to get healthier, we have to send you to another book to learn about what healthy relationships look like and how to get out of unhealthy ones!)

Choosing weight loss surgery to treat the disease of morbid obesity makes logical sense in a number of arenas. That does not translate to anything being easy.

From a physiological perspective, weight loss surgery, in many cases, quickly remits the symptoms of type 2 diabetes. Because weight loss occurs so quickly after WLS, blood pressure often returns to a healthy level in a short period of time, cholesterol levels drop, and the risks of heart disease and stroke are markedly decreased. With rapidly decreasing weight, a person's energy level improves dramatically, which leads to an improved ability to exercise more frequently and with greater intensity—and much less pain! This is a positive energy loop. Weight loss . . . leads to increased energy . . . leads to the ability to exercise more easily . . . leads to increased weight loss . . . *all* leading to better health and an improved quality of life!

Speaking of exercise . . . it *is* one of the necessary lifelong changes that come with weight loss territory. And I don't know many people who would describe exercise as being "easy."

2008 Physical Guidelines for Americans: "To achieve and maintain a healthy body weight, adults should do the equivalent of 150 minutes of moderate-intensity aerobic activity each week. If necessary, adults should increase their weekly minutes of aerobic physical activity gradually over time and decrease calorie intake to a point where they can achieve calorie balance and a healthy weight. Some adults will need a higher level of physical activity than others to achieve and maintain a healthy body weight. Some may need more than the equivalent of 300 minutes per week of moderate-intensity activity." (http://1 .usa.gov/14iTqb).

Although it gets easier to exercise as you lose weight, it sometimes isn't easy, and it doesn't necessarily become something a person *likes* or *looks forward to doing*! For those lucky few who actually do come to love and look forward to exercising (which, I might add, is more than daily *activity* and does involve sweating), the rest of us can struggle through our "love of exercise envy." For those of us—the majority, who don't always look forward to exercising, *but do it anyway*—more power to us! Whether you like exercise or do it even if you don't like it, let me ask: What is easy about exercising? Not much!

Exercise is a commitment those who choose to have weight loss surgery make prior to having surgery.

Exercise is not easy—especially before you lose significant amounts of weight. As already noted—there's nothing easy about weight loss surgery (and the commitments that go with it)!

Remember—there are many things besides exercising that you do nearly every single day that you don't necessarily "like" to do but do anyway: get gas in the car; go through the "get ready for work in the morning" routine of showering, make-up, hair, shaving and whatever else you do before work; return phone calls to people you may not feel like talking to; and pay bills. My reason for bringing this up is because the mindset of "I can't" isn't operated on or removed during weight loss surgery. The truth was, before surgery, "I can't exercise" may have been true! As the weight comes off, your mindset has to be altered just as your clothing size is! Remember that you do all sorts of other things you don't want to do or like to do or that may be "painful," but you have done them for years! Now, you add exercise to that list!

Nope! It's not easy. But it's worth it!

The number one reason (*excuse*) people share with me for not being able to exercise is "I don't have time." I found an incredible quote, spoken by the former prime minister of the United Kingdom, Edward Stanley about exercise and time, which I feel compelled to share with you since I'm on the topic for only a moment: *"Those who think they have no time for bodily exercise will sooner or later have to find time for illness."*

Journals

How about *this* for not easy? Something that improves your follow-through with physical health is to maintain a food diary and an exercise diary. Not easy, but one of the most powerful tools to maximize the effect of weight loss surgery. Food and exercise diaries are essential to sustaining your weight loss. Whether you like to, want to, or feel like it, *maintain food and exercise diaries in order to sustain your weight loss*! Maintaining a food diary is the best way to remain completely honest about the types and quantities of food you eat as well as the frequency of your eating. I'm not talking about counting calories. Is it easy to keep records of what you eat, when you eat, how you feel when you eat? Is it easy to keep records of when you exercise, what type of exercise you chose, and for what period of time you engaged in the exercise? Um… *no*! Successful post-ops do these things because they want to maintain their weight loss.

Psychologically, weight loss surgery increases a person's outlook. For the first time in a long time, WLS people experience *hope*. There is hope that they will see significant weight loss results, *hope* that they will be able to enjoy activities they had, for so long, abandoned. For some, there is *hope* of engaging in activities for the first time. Symptoms of depression often disappear following WLS as these hopes are realized and life becomes increasingly filled with daily activities made easier because of weight loss, and new adventures are sought out and accomplished. A sense of efficacy returns or is developed as people realize, *"I can do this!"* This realization comes with every healthy food choice they make, every active step they take, and with every positive risk that is taken. Self-confidence improves as people lose weight and engage more fully in life. In turn, WLS patients interact with others more confidently.

In addition to the many positive psychological outcomes related to having weight loss surgery, there are times when a person is faced with painful issues related to psychological problems surrounding obesity. Obesity could be the cause of these issues, or the issues may be consequences of obesity. *Facing these issues is not easy. Having weight loss surgery and addressing these issues is not easy.* Again, doing so is definitely worth it! Choosing to deal with these problems can mean the difference between keeping excess weight off and unwanted weight regain.

Research indicates that obese people often struggle with depression, anxiety, have a tendency to express psychological distress through physical complaints, have poor impulse control, low self-esteem, and an impaired quality of life.

Socially, as people lose weight, they are more likely to attend events and social activities they avoided when they were carrying excess weight. They get to attend their kids' school programs, sporting activities, and musical performances and to chaperone field trips. Other adults respond positively in kind to the more outgoing demeanor that weight loss can bring and to a more approachable and healthy person (who brilliantly opted to have weight loss surgery). Sometimes it's upsetting to people who have recently lost weight when those who didn't interact with them when they were at their heaviest suddenly take interest in them. Is it easy for the post-op who was previously shy and "invisible" to others to all of a sudden start taking social risks? As you'll read in the stories that follow, this is definitely not easy for some.

Personal and social relationships change after you have weight loss surgery. The changes that take place in your life, internally and socially, can sometimes be confusing to you, as well as to the people who are closest to you. At times you will be scared about people's reactions to your weight loss. Mad, sad, glad, and scared. You'll feel them all in relation to your weight loss and the changes in your social life. *Not easy.*

Just as you will have emotional reactions to your weight loss, so will family members and friends. Even though they may genuinely be happy for you, they sometimes have emotional reactions none of you anticipate, such as:

- jealousy about the way people look at you after you have lost weight
- envy that they are not getting the same amount of attention as you
- anger because you participate in more social activities as a thin person and are leaving home more often
- fear (on the part of spouses or significant others) that you will become interested in someone else
- irritation as you learn to set healthy boundaries and start saying "no"
- annoyance at your seeming obsession with weight loss issues
- negativity and spite from family members and others for all of the above reasons

The social benefits of losing harmful, excessive weight are numerous and enhance improved personal happiness. Like most other aspects of having weight loss surgery, there are aspects of changing our social relationships following weight loss surgery that can be difficult. *Again—weight loss surgery and the accompanying changes in one's life are not easy!*

The initial weight loss following surgery is *faster* than losing weight without surgery. *Faster does not equate to easy.* In fact, the weight loss happens so rapidly that it can actually be more difficult in some ways to deal with. The mind struggles to keep pace with the body in terms of the changes. Not just the physical changes, although the rapid changes in body size can be a struggle for some. Outside observers are curious to know what is causing the weight loss to happen so quickly—they can't understand how a person can lose so much weight in such a short amount of time. Ironically, these same people often don't understand the causes of obesity, either.

The following poem, submitted by a surgical weight loss patient, makes clear the fact that sustaining weight loss, after surgery or any other means, is not easy:

Some Days It Seems Like I Know Nothing

Patterns from the past keep creeping in

Tough days
Tough weeks

My plans fall short

Patterns creep back in

I have fallen short

I have fallen down in my mind

Food
I don't know how to do it without you

You have been my friend
My friend when I am down

Mind snap back
Snap back now

Don't let me down

Pick up
Listen

Listen we can make this right
The right decision for now

Food
You will no longer be my drug
You will no longer be my friend

I will make this right
I will make the right decision

The right decision now

—Andrew Martin, February 4, 2011

With every day, you have the choice to make the right decision—*now*! Ask yourself in a variety of situations, "What is my role here?" "What is the right decision in this situation?" Remember the recovery slogan:

Always do the next right thing.

(Notice it doesn't say, "Always do the next *easy* thing?" Living a healthy life after weight loss surgery is not easy! Weight loss surgery provides a tool that results in weight coming off quickly and assists a person in eating smaller amounts of food. That is basically it. The person then does the rest—and "the rest" is not easy!

Good news! You don't have to live perfectly! Many people stop eating healthfully or exercising because they don't do it "perfectly." Maybe they miss a day of exercise and the shame of "failure" sets in, so they stop exercising all together. Many times people "cheat" on their diets and fall into the pit of shame, and emotionally beat themselves up for "failing." Rather than start over immediately, they give up. Attempting to be perfect is an impossible task, one that usually leads to an excuse to stop doing "the next right thing." A great blog post from one of the early bloggers in the WLS community writes about perfection and shame:

Do you want to be perfect or happy?
Stop toxic shame.

I recently read an article by Brené Brown (http://bit.ly/lep8wn) who is a research professor at the University of Houston

Graduate College of Social Work. I feel like she lives in my head. The article perfectly describes how so many who have weight loss surgery believe that life will be perfect when . . .

- I lose the weight . . .
- I get that man . . . or that woman.
- I get that job . . .
- I get reconstructive surgery . . .

And yes, I've mentioned all this before but I'm going to say it again. All these things are the greener grass on the other side of the fence. If you are always looking to get to the other side of the fence, you never get there! Even if you do get over the fence, there will just be another fence and another. . . . You never . . . ever . . . get there. So what do you do? You start to look at the things in your life you are fortunate enough to have and you start being grateful. When you covet someone else's "anything" there are just as many people wanting what you have. No matter what your life is like there are hundreds of thousands of people on this earth that would LOVE to be in your shoes. We are generally spending so much time wishing for things we don't have that we never appreciate the things we've got. You may think that's silly and no fun but I believe it's equally silly and no fun to wish for something you don't have.

Many of my blog posts have said how we can ill afford guilt/ blame/shame/judgment, but I love how Ms. Brown points out that we believe perfection will alleviate the pain of those emotions. So, if we understand that perfection is not really possible, and that means we cannot avoid the pain, what do we do to avoid it? We stop doing things that cause the dehumanization of others. We stop actions that make others feel "less than." Forums and Facebook are full of people making others feel "less than" . . . they are full of people dealing out toxic shame.

John Bradshaw wrote a book called *Healing the Shame that Binds You.* He discusses dehumanization or "otheration" (others making you feel less than): "Toxic shame is either inhuman or dehumanizing. The demand for a false self to cover and hide the authentic self necessitates a life dominated by doing and achievement. Everything depends on performance and achievement rather than on being. Being requires no measurement: it is its own justification. Being is grounded in an inner life that grows in richness. Toxic shame looks to the outside for happiness and validation, since the inside is flawed and defective. Toxic shame is spiritual bankruptcy."

Ask yourself the next time you type something or say something about others . . . are you contributing to someone's toxic shame? Remember:

- I am enough . . .
- I AM enough!

I think you are enough, too. Stop toxic shame and we can just be . . . enough.

—Blog post by Yvonne McCarthy (www.wlssuccess.com)

For some people who elect to have weight loss surgery, their lives prior to surgery were far from easy. The next chapter begins with the story by one of the book's contributors. Throughout the story of how she became morbidly obese, she highlights many of the causes of obesity, which are numerous. She knows that life as an obese person is not easy, and she also knows that going through the process of weight loss surgery is not easy. This woman truly understands the difficult and painful contribution that emotional issues play in terms of weight gain.

A Longing

To have a time when food no longer calls
To walk without pain
To run again
To hike without being winded
All these things I want and more

I've heard the work will be worth it
No, I know it will
All I want is not to be stuck
Stuck in a cycle of endless eating

The hope is for the future
It is mine to grab

A life without food calling
No longer hearing its voice
But replaced with one of energy and fight
That is my voice of hope

—Andrew Martin, December 1, 2010

CHAPTER THREE

Causes of Obesity

"I am 46 years old. I'm 5'7". I was born and raised in New Orleans, Louisiana. I am the youngest of four children (one sister and two brothers). I was obese from my mid-teenage years until 2009, when I made the life-changing decision to have gastric bypass surgery.

It almost goes without saying that living in New Orleans involves a more than typical obsession with rich, decadent, high-calorie foods. Seafood gumbo and rice, red beans and sausage with rice, muffaletta sandwich (a decadent combination of Italian cold cuts with cheese and olive salad, dripping with oil on an enormous Italian loaf bread), fried shrimp po boys (sandwich on a French bread loaf, kind of like a hoagie), roast beef po boys dripping with gravy and mayonnaise, doberge cake (icing so sweet it makes my husband's cheeks actually tingle!), king cake (a Mardi Gras traditional cake similar to a cinnamon roll or coffee cake slathered with sugar icing), Popeye's fried chicken . . . the list could go on and on before even MENTIONING the fixation on alcohol! Food and alcohol are the center point for all celebrations and festivals (which happen year round) in New Orleans. So, location was my first contributor to being obese.

My father was an alcoholic. My mother was the most altruistic, kind-natured person I ever knew. She married my father and stayed committed to that relationship and our family with little or no regard for her own needs. That is admirable in a way, but was very enabling in terms of my father's addiction. He was never physically abusive. He almost never missed work. He was a high-functioning alcoholic. However, every evening after work, he would go straight to one of his regular bars and drink until he staggered home at around 10 p.m. My mother would have dinner waiting for him. He would then drink port wine until he fell asleep—usually at the kitchen table.

He was a very unhappy person. He lamented his lack of success in life. He grew up in Los Angeles, but moved to New Orleans after getting discharged from the Army in 1945 to be with his parents, who had moved back to their native city. He would go into these rages about how he hated the city and how everyone was so stupid. He would verbally abuse my mother regularly. I remember hearing the loud arguments and the hurling of unwarranted insults at night. I remember thinking that I was from New Orleans—did that mean I was worthless and stupid?

There was a large gap between my older siblings and myself (about eight years between the third child and myself). So, by age 10, I was the only child living at home. We also had my father's mother living with us. She was a lifelong alcoholic with Alzheimer's (she stopped drinking once she became elderly). Back then they called it being senile. I shared a room with her for several years.

At about age 10, I started to be on a mission to deal with my father and his behavior. I would start calling all his regular bars and ask for him. When he would get on the phone, I would ask if he was coming home soon. I told him we needed him at home, and asked what we would do if we needed the car for an emergency or something. He would come home maybe a little bit earlier on those nights, but not much.

I started to referee my parents' arguments. I became a therapist of sorts, trying to explain to each of them what the other was trying to say; urging them to listen to each other and come to some middle ground. By the time I was 15 or 16, I started to tell my father that he did not deserve my respect when he was drunk. If he came home drunk, I would not talk to him. If he was sober, I would love to talk to him. That didn't work so well either because he didn't drink less, but I tried to stick to that promise.

My mother was very isolated; she had few activities or pleasures of her own, and no friends. Her only outlet was to talk to her sisters on the phone each day for a little while. Dad finally stopped drinking heavily when I was in college. This environment of growing up with an alcoholic parent who was abusive and damaging was another contributor to my being obese.

When I was growing up, many Sundays were spent at my grandmother's house, which was vacant since she lived with us. My parents needed to tend to the property (lawn, leaves, cleaning, etc.). I was usually just bored and underfoot.

There was an older couple that lived across the street. For this writing, I'll call them the Smiths. Mrs. Smith was an invalid. Mr. Smith would be outside in the yard a lot, doing gardening. He also had a shed where he had many fish aquariums and would tinker around with small motors and electronics. My parents would chat with Mr. Smith on a regular basis, and they would encourage me to go visit him while they were busy cleaning or taking care of the grounds.

When I was about eight years old, I had several encounters with Mr. Smith where he sexually molested me. I was a painfully shy and quiet child. I didn't ever throw a tantrum or demand things or attention. I was not a person to challenge authority, especially growing up going to Catholic school. I was respectful to everyone.

I was also very naïve. Mr. Smith would talk to me while he was gardening. I would watch him and maybe help out a little. He would invite me into his shed to show me his fish tanks. One day, he asked me to sit on his lap. He began to caress me and somehow began to fondle my genital area. He would kiss me too. His face was rough with whiskers. He tasted and smelled like cigarettes. I remember that his hands were very rough and tough. He had dirt or grease under his fingernails all the time. He had tattoos on his forearms, from his time in the war. I remember that I didn't like what he was doing to me. However, he would reassure me that it was okay and would whisper to me that it was a good thing. He told me not to tell anyone about it. I remember just being completely silent but wanting it to stop. I wanted to get away.

I don't remember each event clearly; just flashes of memories. Obviously, I would return to see him even after the first encounter, but I don't really know why or how many times. I think part of me liked that he was giving me some attention and affection, but I didn't like it and I wanted to leave. Somehow I eventually just stopped going to visit him. I never told my parents and was very afraid of what had happened. I think I felt ashamed that I let this happen to me. This experience of being sexually molested was another contributor to my being obese.

When I hit puberty and started my period, it became very scary for me because my period was very irregular. I would sometimes go for a couple of months without my period. Eventually, my mother took me to a gynecologist who diagnosed me with polycystic ovarian syndrome (PCOS). He told me that I would most likely not be able to get pregnant and that I should lose weight to improve the situation. PCOS involves a hormonal issue and a condition of insulin resistance, which contributes to weight gain. I was, I think, 17 at the time of the diagnosis, and about 180 pounds. I was so upset by him telling me to lose weight. I took it very personally and was offended. I did not change anything about my eating habits. Being diagnosed with PCOS was another contributor to my being obese.

Most likely as a combination of the factors already mentioned, I was not a social butterfly as a child or teenager. I did not have tons of friends or go to parties. I had one boy in particular that I 'went out with' but it really amounted more to us just talking on the phone every day. He would come over sometimes and we would sneak to 'make out.' He was a healthy teenage boy, and was definitely interested in 'going all the way,' but I always prevented that. I know that was the right decision and do not claim that it is because of my obesity or low self-esteem. However, I 'broke up' with him and didn't have any other steady boyfriends for the rest of high school.

There was another adult male that I became close to, who also tried very hard to get me to have sex with him. He invited me to his apartment one day and had me pinned down on his bed. After my protests, he did not force me. He wasn't a bad guy either, but should have known better than to try that with a teenage girl. Another time my (much) older sister's boyfriend cornered me when no one else was around and started groping and kissing me. I had to push him off and get away. Again, I never told anyone at the time that these things were happening to me.

I came to the conclusion that men were out for one thing, and they usually did not treat women with love and respect. I think I just decided that I would not find happiness or comfort from relationships with men. I think subconsciously I ate to make myself less attractive to men so I would not have to be bothered with it. I believe that the lack of learning about loving and respectful intimate relationships while I was growing up was a contributor to my being obese.

Money was tight growing up. I saw how my mother struggled to keep it all together. I never demanded things like new clothes or toys or personal items. I used to not even tell my mother if I felt sick because I didn't want them to have to pay for a doctor. We had roaches in our house and could not afford to have pest control. It wasn't unbearable, though. We would go on road trip vacations now and then. Of course, I would end up being in the mature 'adult' role, facilitating my parents' fights or helping to take care of my mother, who would have bathroom accidents due to her constant anxiety and having irritable bowel syndrome. My father's personality and rages dictated how things went for us, and it was not easy to have a fun or relaxed time.

Growing up with these experiences, I became determined to do well in school so that I could get a good job in order to support myself. I would never allow myself to become dependent on any man for support. I would be able to pay for whatever I needed or wanted. And that included whatever food I wanted to eat.

As a teenager, I would relish any opportunity I would have to 'eat out,' which was definitely not fine dining. I would sometimes be able to eat at McDonald's or have other fast food. When I got a part-time job at the mall, I would love to be able to go to lunch in the mall with my own money and sometimes even eat in the sit-down restaurant at the mall. Food was my pleasure, and it would always be there for me. I was so happy that I was able to be in a position to pay for it myself and do what I wanted to make me happy. My experience of doing 'without' important things was another contributor to my being obese.

I went to Catholic school from kindergarten through 12th grade. I am so grateful that my parents invested that money so I would get a better education since the public school system in New Orleans was not up to par with what the private schools could provide. We considered ourselves to be a Catholic family, but we never went to church. I only attended mass when I was at school. When I was an early teenager, I would sometimes go to church on Sunday myself since it was so close to my house.

I feel that I benefitted from learning about Christianity and have always tried to be a Christian person. However, I began to see multiple examples of hypocrisy that I could not ignore within the Catholic faith and in my church parish in particular. One of the main issues I experienced more than once was that some of the people that were in positions of authority in the church and school were typically not good people, but would strut around boldly at Church, pretending to be such good Christian people. I became alienated from the Church after witnessing numerous hypocritical events and also after being disillusioned about how Jesus or God would 'allow' these things and other bad things to happen to good people. I felt like many people used organized religious services more to uphold their reputations to friends, neighbors, family, clients, etc. than to sincerely seek to participate in a service to serve others and reflect on how to maintain and improve their Christian behaviors. I also felt like many other people used organized religion as a crutch to abdicate any personal responsibility for their own choices and to pray for everything from a cure to a disease, to a better job, to a better marriage.

I could not find comfort or fulfillment from my religion and was more interested in getting away from what I thought was inappropriate, insincere, and hypocritical behavior. Therefore, the lack of a spiritual harmony was another contributor to my being obese.

It was my senior year in high school when I met my future husband while working at the mall. He was a super nice guy. He asked me to go on what essentially was a 'pity date' to his family party for Christmas Eve. He asked me to go so that he would have a girl with him. So, I went as a favor to him. He asked me to go out for New Year's Eve to a friend's house, and I said yes. He was so nice. He was not trying to grope me. We started going to movies or out to eat more often. That fall I was going to college, which was about 90 minutes from home. We continued to be friends and go out as a group with my girlfriends. Again, there was no sexual pressure, and he treated me with respect. We officially started 'going out,' and we dated all through college.

We got married after college, and things were good. He was also overweight, and we both happily enjoyed our freedom of being able to eat out all the time and get fast food whenever we wanted it. However, the marriage wasn't completely perfect.

The intimacy was not normal or very frequent. I assumed it was because I was so unattractive and fat. I just figured he didn't want to be intimate with me. That feeling of rejection caused me to eat even more to get comfort. I was up to 250 pounds. After a couple of years, I found some items in our home that led me to suspect that he was homosexual. I confronted him and he vehemently denied it. He went to counseling, which did not help.

This problem became worse and worse over time, and with his denials, led me to believe more and more that I was undesirable. I tried to learn about how to be a better sexual partner. I bought books and instructional tapes. I encouraged him to watch them with me. We had a romantic retreat where I basically jumped him in an effort to improve our intimacy. By some miracle, I ended up pregnant.

Our son was born, and we focused on parenting. My husband was the best father. Everyone thought we had the perfect marriage. No one knew what it was really like. By this time, I had tried Jenny Craig and lost about 70 pounds. I used to reward myself after each weigh in by getting a Quarter Pounder with Cheese value meal! Needless to say, I gained it all back plus more. When my son was still a baby, we started individual and couples counseling. I finally realized my husband was homosexual and was not able to admit it. I decided to stay in the marriage for the sake of my son. I became more and more depressed, and continued to use food to comfort myself. Finally, when my son was about six years old, I chose to divorce my husband. It took a lot of courage. However, I still did not address this issue of my low self-esteem, which was a serious contributor to my being obese.

After my divorce, I began to realize that all men do not just want skinny women. I began to understand that many men actually prefer larger women. I started to date different men, but tried to keep a distance so that I would not get burned again. I tried different diets but was unsuccessful. I worked with nutritionists, joined gyms, hired personal trainers, and bought home exercise equipment and tapes. But I never really stopped being a person that was unfulfilled and continued to use food to try to make me happy.

They say that many obese people are constantly trying to please others. They try to avoid conflict and want to be accepted. They take care of everyone else's needs before they worry about their own needs. All of these things were true about me. But I was trying to continue with long-term therapy to work on making myself healthier.

About nine years ago, not long after my divorce, I made an online male friend. He was so nice to chat with, and we shared lots of things in common, both of us having grown up in New Orleans. He asked me out numerous times, but I would decline, saying I was not interested in a serious relationship. I finally said yes to one of his invitations, and it changed my life. He and I quickly connected in a truly respectful, loving, and mutually beneficial relationship. We have been married now for six years. This man loves me for who I am on the inside and outside. We spend so much of our time trying to make sure we are doing things for each other. He says I have an 'old soul'—that I am one of the few remaining women that isn't self-absorbed or selfish and demanding. I don't know that I'm only one of a few women like that, but I feel the same about him. He is so respectful and thoughtful. We tell each other we love each other probably a dozen times a day. We call each other regularly during each day when at work, etc. We can't wait to see each other.

We have a great intimate relationship and have regular date night on Fridays. It isn't completely perfect, as no marriage is perfect. His moods still sometimes affect me and how my day goes. With all my issues of growing up with an abusive, angry father, I still cringe any time there is any anger on his part about anything. However, I am working on that with my therapist to not take it so personally and to not let it affect me so badly.

As my marriage provided me with more and more personal satisfaction, emotional fulfillment, and stability, I began to explore ways to finally get control of my obesity. I started to research weight loss surgery when my employer's insurance announced it would start to cover the procedure. I researched extensively. I read four or five books on the subject. I met with the surgeon. I decided I would try the six-month supervised diet required by the insurance company and would see how I would do. I was very successful on that diet, losing about 45 pounds. I decided I would defer the decision to have the surgery to see if I could maintain the weight loss on my own.

Right about that time, my father's health started to decline dramatically. My mother had died ten years earlier, but my father had been very independent and self-sufficient up until this point. My siblings and I realized that we needed to intervene, and it quickly escalated to an extended period of time where I was heavily involved with my father's care. That included dealing with his negative and abusive personality up close again. I continued to do my best to help him, including dealing with difficult family dynamics because it was the right thing to do.

However, I quickly reverted back to eating to comfort myself during this stressful period. I would drop my father off at his assisted living home, and drive straight to McDonald's for a double Quarter Pounder with Cheese, super-sized fries, and large chocolate shake. And, more than once, the shake machine would be broken. I was so angry! I actually called McDonalds' customer service line to complain. I was sitting in my car in the McDonald's parking lot, on my cell phone screaming at the representative that they just did NOT understand that I NEEDED that shake, and it was not there for me.

Needless to say, my weight crept back up again, now to 288. I was five pounds away from my heaviest of 293 after all that work to get the weight off. I told myself I would start on Monday to diet and exercise. I was wasting a lot of money on a gym membership that I never used. I was on two prescription medicines for high blood pressure. I was on an antidepressant for migraines. I had sleep apnea and had a CPAP machine to use when I slept. I was getting knee pain and feared a knee replacement was in my near future. I told myself that I would start again on Monday—over and over again, and each Monday would not become THAT Monday. I felt so sad. I felt like such a failure to have allowed myself to gain all that weight back.

One day I was in bed, lying awake before the alarm went off—again—since I was so stressed out. I considered what it would take for me to stick with the plan to start dieting and exercising. How could I convince myself to get control of it? Suddenly, I decided that the best way for me to stay committed to losing weight and keeping it off was to go ahead and get the weight loss surgery. I knew what I was getting into. I felt it was safe, and not 'too drastic' anymore, considering my inability to control my weight so many times. If I invested all that time and money into having the surgery, it would be enough to force me to stay committed to it and to not let it be another failed diet attempt.

That was it! I would do it. I would be making a very serious, permanent life decision to make myself healthier. Right then, during that 10- or 15-minute period of time as I thought it over, a strong sense of peace came over me. It was like I experienced immense relief. I just knew it was time for me to go ahead with the surgery. I felt completely calm and happy with my decision. I didn't tell my family right away, but I scheduled my appointment with the surgeon to begin the pre-surgery testing. Then, I let my family and close friends know about my decision. Everyone was supportive of my decision.

On June 25, 2009, I had the gastric bypass surgery. I have
had no complications from the surgery, and have worked very
hard to stick with the program of eating right, cooking healthier,
exercising regularly, participating in online support, reading bariatric books and articles, and continuing my therapy to address
emotional and behavioral issues. I have lost 150 pounds in about
18 months, and am so happy with my decision. I feel like I will
be a long-term success, due to my strong desire to make the
permanent life changes needed so I can maintain my health.

Wow! This woman knows the causes of her obesity, which are
complicated and numerous. Her story shows the willingness it
takes to identify your personal issues and the tremendous courage it takes to address them. She continues in personal therapy
to work on the issues from her past that collectively resulted in
her being emotionally dependent on food to avoid dealing with
unpleasant feelings related to emotional pain. Along with some
medical problems, being raised in an environment that focused on
food, and having experienced verbal, emotional, sexual, and vicarious abuse (which means witnessing someone else being abused),
this woman became obese. She very wisely knew that, while weight
loss surgery would help her to lose her excess weight, unless she
worked through the emotional issues that resulted in her overeating unhealthy food and ultimately screaming at a customer service employee at a fast food restaurant because she "needed that
shake," she would likely return to emotional eating. She knew her
obesity was a symptom of the real problem, and the importance of
addressing the issues underneath the emotional eating.

Weight loss surgery does not result in losing the desire to eat
when one is stressed, angry, sad, lonely, depressed, scared, exhil-
arated, or bored. Weight loss surgery does not stop emotional
eating. That takes the help of others. Depending on the issues
involved, professional therapists are usually the best ones to help
people work through issues that are related to emotional eating.

In the professional continuing education programs I present to medical and mental health care professionals, I discuss the causes of obesity noted in the professional literature. The most common factors associated with the causes of obesity include:

- Genetics
  - Continued scientific studies do link obesity with genetics. To what extent genetics are "responsible" for obesity is still unknown. Suffice it to say that there is little denial that to some degree, the *tendency* for obesity is genetic.

- Environment
  - Ask anyone over the age of 40 how often their family ate their evening meal at a restaurant, and they will probably indicate that eating out was a rare occasion reserved for special events. Today, some people may think holidays are the only time you use the kitchen in your house!
  - If you've ever heard me speak, I've probably mentioned the poem by Dorothy Law Nolte called "Children Learn What They Live." The kinds of food your children eat are something they learn, in large part, from their parents. If you have all sorts of junk food around your house and there are no guidelines about when or how much of it people can eat, your kids are going to adopt the attitude that all forms of junk food are allowed at any time. If you prepare white rice, noodles, and potatoes with gravy and butter for most meals, your children will learn to consume simple carbs (which have very limited amounts of nutritional value) on a regular basis. If you use whole grain breads, whole grain pasta, and brown rice, your family will learn to eat these healthier varieties of carbohydrates. If you allow a limited number of snacks, which are chosen for their nutritional value, then your kids will learn to snack on fruits, nuts, and yogurt. If you opt to have a non-nutritious snack or dessert from time to time, they will realize that these sorts of food are reserved for occasional consumption.

- Metabolism
  - The Centers for Disease Control and Prevention define metabolic rate as "The rate at which the body uses energy. When measured while a person is at rest, the resulting value represents the lowest (i.e., basal) rate of energy expenditure necessary to maintain basic body functions." In other words, the basal metabolic rate determines how many calories your body needs simply to keep itself functioning—breathing, pumping blood through your system, and maintaining your body's temperature. Resting metabolic rate can vary substantially from one person to the next. This can help to explain why some people gain weight more easily than others and tend to have more difficulty losing weight.

- Culture
  - Obesity is truly a worldwide epidemic. In all cultures, as noted by the World Health Organization, "there has been: an increased intake of energy-dense foods that are high in fat, salt, and sugars but low in vitamins, minerals, and other micronutrients; and a decrease in physical activity due to the increasingly sedentary nature of many forms of work, changing modes of transportation, and increasing urbanization."

- Illness/Medication
  - There are some illnesses and medications that do cause weight gain. Some health conditions associated with hormones can cause weight gain. Hypothyroidism, Cushing's syndrome, and polycystic ovarian syndrome (PCOS) are examples.

  - Certain medications are also associated with weight gain. Steroids, in particular, can result in a weight gain ranging from a few pounds to 100 pounds or more. Other medications that have been linked to weight gain include antidepressants, antipsychotics, antiseizure medications, diabetes medications, high blood pressure medications, and heartburn medications. For some women, the birth control pill can be associated with weight gain, although the increased weight may be related to fluid retention.

- Age
  - As we get older, we tend to *lose muscle,* especially if we're less active. Muscle loss can slow down the rate at which your body burns calories.
  - Did you know:
    - American adults experience gradual decrease in muscle tissue at the *approximate rate of six pounds of muscle loss per decade.*
    - Americans experience a gradual decrease in resting metabolism *of approximately 3 percent metabolic rate reduction per decade.*
    - Weight gain may underestimate fat gain by up to 50 percent due to unrecognized muscle loss.

- Lack of Sleep
  - Studies show that the risk of gaining more than 50 pounds is increased by 50 percent when people get five hours of sleep or less per night.
  - Studies find that the less people sleep, the more likely they are to be overweight or obese. It's also been shown that *70 percent of sleep apnea patients are obese.* Part of the reason that people who sleep fewer hours are heavier is they seem to prefer foods that are higher in calories and carbohydrates, which can lead to over-eating, weight gain, and obesity. Hormones that are released during sleep control appetite and the body's use of energy. If a person doesn't get enough sleep, these body functions can become unbalanced, and can result in weight gain.

- Psychological Factors
  - Research indicates that obese people often struggle with depression or anxiety, have a tendency to express psychological distress through physical complaints, have poor impulse control or low self-esteem, and have an impaired quality of life.

There are clearly numerous interacting factors that play a part in a person becoming obese. We have very little influence over many of these things. For example, our genetics are what they are. Some medical conditions are beyond our control. Many of the causes of obesity, however, are things over which we have some influence. We cannot control or change our age, but we can maximize our body's functioning by remaining active and involved in healthy behaviors. There are factors we have considerable influence over. We can most often choose if we get enough sleep or not. If we have psychological issues negatively affecting our weight, we have the option of seeking help for them and learning more effective ways to deal with issues without using food or other substances or behaviors that cause more problems and often jeopardize our health.

Weight loss surgery doesn't change one's age or genetics or the people and problems in a person's life. However, anyone can utilize the services of mental health professionals and other support people to assist them in learning effective tools to use in dealing with issues that are related to weight gain.

My very good friend, the Bariatric Guru (Erin Akey, founder of the Bariatric Breakthrough Challenge), speaks regularly about post-ops needing to take responsibility for their personal choices after weight loss surgery. I agree. People who choose to have weight loss surgery have a responsibility to get help for those causes of their obesity that weight loss surgery cannot positively impact. If they do not, they stand a good chance of regaining weight following the surgery. As was stated in Chapter One: "Having weight loss surgery is not easy." In fact, taking responsibility to deal with the issues contributing to one's obesity can be downright hard! But, oh—so worth it!

The life of an obese person is often not an easy one, just as weight loss surgery is not an easy venture. In the next chapter, we hear from people about the reality of their lives as obese children and adults.

CHAPTER FOUR

Life as an Obese Person

What's it like to live as an obese person? In a poignant narrative, this contributor describes what many obese patients experience:

"Being overweight, in my family, is a legacy. And it is a legacy that goes back many, many generations. Before I went to school, I really wasn't aware I was fat. There were signs (such as nicknames like 'Butterball' from my family members) and one of my grandmothers who would comment on 'How BIG you are!' which should have made me understand. She would often comment on what I was eating, and whether or not I should be eating 'anything at your size'. Despite these signs, I had a great childhood with my nuclear family, and some extended family members, where I was nurtured and loved.

However, I was often nurtured with food. Because being overweight was historically something accepted in my family, there didn't always seem to be an emphasis on weight or health. But it would wax and wane, with my mother's efforts to lose weight. When she would get on a diet craze, she would bring the whole family along with her. Primarily, we did Weight Watchers as this was my mother's dieting plan of choice. Despite multiple attempts at participation in this program over many different times, we never did active things as a family, even though Weight Watchers encouraged activity. We did camp, and go fishing, and go hunting—but we didn't go on walks, or participate in sports, or do any other active things. Nor were active things encouraged.

My thoughts on this: my father worked a labor-intensive job that required 10 to 12 hours of work each day and often included weekends. He was fairly active, though overweight, but he was tired when he did have time off, and he didn't realize that exercise would help him feel less fatigue rather than more.

Again, obesity is a generational issue in my family. My mother was a stay-at-home mom and has always preferred more sedentary activities, like reading, crafting, etc. These activities were encouraged, particularly in my case because I was academically advanced for my age. However, even though more cerebral activities were the norm, I did have opportunities to participate in ballet and T-ball and gymnastics. Unfortunately, my weight would often prevent me from succeeding in those types of activities, and it would further discourage me and push me back toward reading, crafting, and other sedentary activities where I felt comfort and joy, rather than failure.

My temperament is one of sensitivity—or perhaps more correctly—oversensitivity. I believe this is my temperament, and my propensity to be oversensitive was exacerbated by ridicule from peers while participating in school, sports, and other extracurricular activities.

One particular situation that resonates as an 'aha moment' in my life began in second grade. Our elementary school (one of three in a small, rural town in eastern Washington state) was unique in that first- through third-grades were all in a large room with six different classrooms sectioned off with cubicle-type walls, bookshelves, and chalkboards. As a result of the close proximity of all of the students, all of the grades would often participate in activities together. During one of these all-inclusive activities, we were working on health. They herded each of us down the hall to the scale, much like you would see in movies about new military recruits going through processing.

I fretted the whole time down the line, as I waited my fate. I knew that I would be the fattest kid in class, and I had already learned to avoid the scale by this age. Each student would get weighed, and then the teacher would record the weight on his chart. By the time it was my turn, the teacher had said very little other than 'Go here,' etc. He gave instructions quietly while getting the task done. When it was my turn, I jumped on the scale in haste, thinking that the faster I did this, the better off I would be and that it couldn't accurately read my weight if I hurried.

This magical thinking didn't work, and the scale registered—211 pounds.

I was eight years old. Unlike for the other students, my weight was not simply recorded. The teacher screamed out (I am not exaggerating this part in any way, shape or form), 'WOW, 211 pounds! That's a lot!' All of the other students, who were following instructions and standing close to the weigh-in area, heard him. I know this due to the cacophony of sound as people discussed my weight, my disgusting existence, my lack of willpower, my inability to be 'cool'— all the things that first-through-third-graders find important. And the ridicule didn't stop there. I was ridiculed for many years. I went to school with many of my classmates from kindergarten until graduation (probably close to 80 percent of them). New students would be told of this experience as though it was news that was commensurate with the state of the union, acid rain, and what clothes were considered cool to wear (all topics of vital importance back in those days).

School was always a place where I got the most ridicule. I struggled quite a bit and internalized the hateful and traumatizing things that were said about me or directly to me. As a result, I would do anything in my power to appear cool or good. I wasn't above lying about something cool I was going to do, or exaggerating capabilities, etc. I needed to PROVE to everyone that I had worth. Luckily, teachers gave me approval, particularly because I was well behaved and academically gifted. However, the more I lied and exaggerated with my peers, the worse my relationships became with them.

A second situation that was difficult for me was in the sixth grade. Many of the girls in my class (who were also in my Campfire group, T-ball team, etc.) sent me a letter and they told me how much they hated me, how much they hated my lying, bragging, and sucking up to the teachers, and most importantly how much they hated me for being fat. They all signed it and told me that they weren't going to acknowledge my existence (I paraphrase here) because fat people were worthless and weren't worth their time.

There were two other girls in the class that didn't participate. They were the other outcasts—ones who were also overweight and ones who were very poor. They were the only people who would talk to me and for that, I will be forever grateful. Beth and Patty, you know who you are, and if you ever read this please know that you saved my life. Without you I would have killed myself, because that is when the thoughts of suicide began.

Despite this, I tried to participate in activities in school. I fell on a girl in volleyball, and hurt her leg. I don't think she has ever forgiven me for this, because she wouldn't even acknowledge me at our 20-year class reunion, and we went through K through 12 together. I was a Campfire member, and stayed involved until I got my WO-HE-LO medallion (comparable to the Eagle Scout award for Boy Scouts). It became my goal, consciously or unconsciously, to be the best and smartest in the class. I thought if I did something outright that showed my worth and I got approval for it, that it would help me. Being the smartest just further ostracized me, unless I was willing to do homework for the popular kids (which I admit to doing in hopes of getting back into the circle of friends I once enjoyed).

During my entire school years, I would yo-yo with weight. When I was thinner, I was given more approval. I was treated better by teachers, retailers, and nearly everyone when I was thinner. And when I gained weight, I would hear, 'You would be so pretty if you only lost weight. What's wrong with you?' By then there was so much psychologically wrong with me that it would take much more than what this book affords time to explain. Suffice it to say that by age 16, I considered suicide and spent time in a psychiatric facility for three days. I started therapy. And I would continue to yo-yo.

In college, I managed four years of healthy eating and exercise. I drank instead. I quit drinking because 'good girls' and people who were going to become psychologists weren't supposed to have addictions. Little did I realize that food was my addiction, because like alcohol, it shielded me from emotions which were difficult for me to handle.

I went through many boyfriends, seeking approval. I married someone the first time because he was from high school and that represented 'approval' from a group that ostracized me and hated me. It only lasted two years. I went through many other relationships, some from the Internet, some from the local town, but usually it was because I would easily have sex, thinking this was a sign from the man that he 'loved' me or 'approved' of me. Despite having a master's degree in psychology, I couldn't see what I was doing. I didn't care—because I needed approval. And I needed food. It became how I dealt with all things.

Eventually, I met and married someone who loved me despite my size and doted on me. We shared similar ideations about life, and I had grown quite a bit in psychological ways. He treated me well, despite my weight. However, my weight was still an issue for me. After we got pregnant, the weight was super-important again. Being 400 pounds and trying to have a child was danger-ous for us both. It was dangerous and complicated. But, I had him and added him to our family, which included my older boy from my first marriage.

My youngest was born with a neuronal migration malforma-tion, which may or may not be due to my weight. As I have so many times before, I internalized his illness as my fault. But, I used my guilt and shame to find him the best treatment possible. They told us that he wouldn't live to be older than age two. In ret-rospect, that's when I gave up totally on my weight and health. I hated me and I ate all the emotions away. And then, he was five. I realized that he was going to be okay, because the doc-tors continuously told us that he was a 'miracle' and would live a primarily normal life with a normal longevity.

I didn't put this together until after I started seeing a thera-pist and preparing for weight loss surgery, but the horrible and excessive bingeing and restricting I was doing after my youngest child's birth was punishment for my existence and for potentially being the cause of his issues. That's when the weight started to come off—I was 623 pounds at my highest weight in 2008. When I started the weight loss surgery program with my insur-ance company in May 2009, I was down to 471. I had surgery on March 22, 2010, and weighed 434 that day. I now weigh 179.

No weight is going to make me happy—I have to make me happy. I have to deal with emotions—good, difficult, or indifferent. I have forgiven my past. And I have forgiven me. My existence is something I no longer apologize for, but I do thank my Creator daily for giving me life and giving me the power to learn from my past, adjust to changes and transitions, and learn that emotions won't kill me, but eating them away most certainly will."

Families often have obesity that goes back many generations. Until someone makes a dramatic change in behaviors, that "family legacy of obesity" is certain to continue. Familial obesity is likely a combination of genetics, learned behavior, and poor health habits. Remember, children *do* learn what they live. If you come from generations where obesity is the norm in your family, being the person who chooses to have weight loss surgery makes you a pioneer! True pioneers didn't just make their way across the landscape, they dealt with issues they encountered along the way. Therefore, if you are the weight loss trailblazer in your family, be sure to truly show the way to improved health and a better quality of life: address the issues surrounding your obesity. If that means seeing a nutritionist to learn how to read food labels, do it. If it means having the nutritionist take you on an educational tour of the grocery store to learn about finding the healthiest foods, then do it. If it means hiring a personal trainer, then do that. If it means seeing a minister or a therapist to work through the hurt and pain associated with having been obese or on issues that preceded your obesity, then do it. If you need to learn to set goals and have some-one urge you to complete them, hire a life coach. Whatever you need to do, do it! Break the chain of obesity in your family. What a legacy that would be!

Name-calling is, sadly, something most obese people suffer through at some point. Whether the names come from family members, peers, teachers, coaches, or bullies—it hurts. I've often thought about the saying, "Stick and stones will break your bones, but words will never hurt you." What sort of imbecile was the per-son who came up with that one? I think it should go like this: "Sticks and stones can break your bones, but words can *really* hurt you—for a long damn time!"

People have an amazing ability to recall, with great detail, times during which someone said something hurtful or cruel to them. Who said it, where it took place, what they were wearing . . . I've heard numerous such stories. Most important is how you felt in response to the name-calling.

Those feelings are buried deep within you. It's great to get them out, simply by telling someone in as much detail as you can about the situation. Here's a secret—when you tell someone the detailed story, you'll be feeling those feelings like you experienced them at the age you were when the situation took place. So don't be surprised if you feel them intensely, or if you have some fear about allowing yourself to let them resurface! Take the plunge—allow yourself to feel them, to share them, and to talk about them. Then you can move on. I promise you'll feel "lighter"!

And then, of course, there are the well-intentioned "suggestions" from loved ones and strangers alike. "Do you think you should really eat that?" Lots of folks, as mentioned above, are "often nurtured with food," or forced to eat everything on their plate.

Mother issues, sad to say, frequently have an impact on a child's relationship with food, as noted by this book contributor: *"When she would get on a diet craze, she would bring the whole family along with her."* A parent (whether a mom or dad) who regularly goes on and off diets, particularly if the person makes yo-yo dieting a "family affair," fails to teach kids to eat healthy on a consistent basis. If a parent laments about personal weight and body imperfections, or vocalizes dieting "failures" in front of their children, the kids learn to emphasize appearance and to judge themselves based on their weight or body proportions. This can lead to a negative body image and disordered eating. It also teaches "stinking thinking," which means, in a word, negativity.

Horrendous stories about kids being weighed and measured in front of the entire class never cease to amaze me. If that weren't bad enough, the stories often include some insensitive, asinine adult who blurts out the child's weight in front of everyone and adds a commentary as well: "WOW, 211 pounds! That's a lot!"

School zones . . . *not* the safety zone they would like to promote themselves as being: *"School was always a place where I got the most ridicule. I struggled quite a bit and internalized the hateful and traumatizing things that were said about me or directly to me. As a result, I would do anything in my power to appear cool or good."* This, too, is an oft-heard refrain from the obese and formerly obese. In an attempt to "appear cool," many overweight or obese kids have done things against their personal values.

Behavior is driven by needs—the need for acceptance may be greater than the need to be true to self. Sadly, this is how so many people "lose" their genuine selves as they become obese. *Recovering* from obesity means, in part, finding out who your authentic self is, and then acting according to your own values, regardless of what other people think or how other people feel.

The contributor above experienced the type of bullying in which she was not only rejected, but told directly by the bullies that *"fat people were worthless and weren't worth their time."* These messages don't fade away just because people get older. The emotional damage caused by these kinds of messages lives on inside a person. Tragically, people often begin to tell themselves the same things through their negative self-talk. (You may have said something like this: "I'm not worth it." "Who would want to be with someone like me?" "I'm so fat/ugly/worthless/lazy, " etc., etc., etc.)

Weight loss surgery does not involve these mental messages being extracted by the surgeon. It takes talking about, maybe even crying and yelling about, the pain of such experiences and resultant self-loathing, with a trusted friend, spiritual adviser, or trained therapist to work through these damaging judgments. And it requires a great deal of changing one's self-talk.

Many obese people work diligently to excel at something in order to attain recognition. *"It became my goal, consciously or unconsciously, to be the best and smartest in the class. I thought if I did something outright that showed my worth and I got approval for it, that it would help me."* And it does help. It helps to be recognized for good grades or musical talent or writing skills or artistic talent when people feel badly about their weight. But it still hurts to be ostracized for your weight. And it can be confusing and maddening when there is fluctuation in weight that is equaled by fluctuation in acceptance:

"When I was thinner, I was given more approval. I was treated better by teachers, retailers, and nearly everyone when I was thinner. And when I gained weight, I would hear, "You would be so pretty if you only lost weight. What's wrong with you?" This contributor bravely acknowledged, *"By then there was so much psychologically wrong with me. . . . "*

How could anyone *not* experience psychological pain when being called names, when being excluded from events and peer groups, when being bullied and humiliated? More courage spoken by this formerly obese person: *"Suffice it to say that by age 16, I considered suicide and spent time in a psychiatric facility for three days. I started therapy."* I applaud her for crying out for help in the only way many adolescents know how. I applaud her for getting therapy. I applaud her for sharing with you how badly she had been hurt and for getting the help she needed.

I thank her profusely for sharing what she shared next: *"In college, I managed four years of healthy eating and exercise. I drank instead. . . . little did I realize that food was my addiction, because like alcohol, it shielded me from emotions which were difficult for me to handle."* The transfer of harmful behavior (from overeating to drinking or to excessive shopping or to gambling or to "sleeping around") is a common occurrence but not commonly understood or acknowledged.

She noted another way she transferred her negative behavior of using food by stating, *"I went through many boyfriends, seeking approval. . . . I would easily have sex, thinking this was a sign from the man that he 'loved' me or 'approved' of me. Despite having a master's degree in psychology, I couldn't see what I was doing. I didn't care—because I needed approval. And I needed food. It became how I dealt with all things."* Again, I say a very heartfelt "thank you" to this brave woman for her honesty and her courage.

My hope is that others reading this book who have felt the need for approval or "love" so strongly that they "don't care" if they violate their own personal codes of conduct will find the courage to heal their wounds in a healthy way.

Our needs drive our behavior. The bottom line is this: food, alcohol, shopping, sex, gambling, Internet, video games . . . you name it . . . none of these things can meet our needs for love, acceptance, approval, or belonging. We can learn to get those needs met in healthy ways and don't have to violate our values. When we go against our own values, we increase the shame we were working to escape. When we learn to meet our emotional needs in healthy ways, then we increase our love for ourselves, along with our self-confidence, our self-esteem, and our self-efficacy.

What a beautiful outcome for this woman who was willing to get the help she needed to work through her issues so that she is able to live without using food to meet her emotional needs and no longer needs a substitute for food in which to hide: *"No weight is going to make me happy—I have to make me happy. I have to deal with emotions—good, difficult, or indifferent. I have forgiven my past. And I have forgiven me. My existence is something I no longer apologize for, but I do thank my Creator daily for giving me life and giving me the power to learn from my past, adjust to changes and transitions, and learn that emotions won't kill me, but eating them away most certainly will."*

Her Day

Everything is a reminder
A reminder of her weight

She starts her day with clothes
It leads to despair
Just another reminder

Then breakfast
It is feared
If she starts, will she stop
She fears food
Another reminder

Going to work
Like a child in a schoolyard
Taunted by the remarks of others
Yet another reminder

While at work
She can be doubted
Is it because of her weight?
She wonders
I have to work harder
She thinks to herself
Reminder after reminder

Now Lunch
It's a break from work
Food will help her cope
She sits staring at her food
She is afraid to eat
It's a reminder

On her way home on the bus
She wonders what others are saying
As her lap hangs over onto the next seat
Are they staring at me?

Finally at home
Food is calling loudly now
A refuge from the day
Able to eat alone
Finding comfort from each bite she eats
But still a reminder

Despair creeps in as the day ends
and the thought of another day is looming

A full day of reminders of the weight she is in

—Andrew Martin, April 11, 2011

The young man in the following story shares the pain of being an obese child. He suffered from teasing by peers and from his family.

He endured social isolation and bruised self-esteem. At a young age, he had weight loss surgery. He now has his entire adult life to have what he notes every overweight person wants—to be healthy.

"I am 20 years old. I have been overweight all my life. In third grade I weighed between 170 and 180 pounds. I was always teased about my weight while I was growing up. I would be in class and hear the kids around me call me names and talk about me behind my back.

Even some family members have teased me about my weight. It's hard to go to school and be teased and then have some family member tease you also. Home is one place you are supposed to feel safe. I've been called Fat Butt, Tubby, Chunky Monkey, Fat Albert, Peter Griffin, etc. You name it, I have been called it. The problem with people is they think, 'Hey I'm not hurting anyone, so what's the big deal?' Well, they don't know that name-calling and teasing hurts emotionally and sometimes physically. The person they pick on may have been dealing with being overweight since childhood.

When I was in the third grade, my family and I went out for some Mexican food one day after school. I choked on a chip, and it was the scariest thing I have ever experienced in my life. I quit eating for a period of four months. All I would eat was ice cream and drink sweet tea. In those four months, I went from being 180 pounds to weighing just 90 pounds. I remember it as if it was just yesterday.

I was working with my dad. He cut yards for a living and had his own lawn business. I was with him and I was really weak. We were cutting the yard of a lady who happened to be an RN. She told my dad, 'This child is dehydrated, and his eyes are in the back of his head. Get him to the ER quickly.' So my dad called my mom, and they took me to the hospital, where they quickly admitted me and started giving me IV fluids. I was in the hospital for two or more days.

My mom and her co-workers encouraged me to eat. When I did eat, it was a bite of ice cream and a taste of a banana. The hospital released me and ordered me to see a lady who would teach me 'how to eat again' and that 'eating was safe.' She got me to eat a banana. After that I stopped seeing her.

I ended up going back to the same Mexican restaurant where

I choked on the chip. The waiter there offered me five dollars to eat a beef burrito. I started eating again. Man, oh, man, did I ever start eating again. I gained all my weight back plus more, when I could have kept it off.

Growing up as an overweight child hurts. I mean, you look at someone who is normal sized and wish you could do half the things they do—like run, ride on rides at fairs or amusement parks, etc. The most hurtful thing is that you are considered unhealthy. The other people aren't. You may even eat the same things they do and even though they don't gain a pound, you do.

It's also hard to make friends and have relationships when you are overweight. I did have friends and a few best friends. My best friends growing up were a male and a female. We could talk about anything. They saw me for me and did not judge me for my size. They saw me as a regular person and not just another fat kid wanting friends. I was shy growing up, which also made it harder to make friends, because I would only talk to people I knew. Most of the time, if you had a class with me you could hear me breathe—that's how shy and quiet I was.

Growing up, I did not do many extracurricular activities or social activities. I did not play any sports for a team. I did not like to go to the dances at school. I liked baseball growing up and wrestling too. I just never chose to participate in them. If I got a chance to play baseball or basketball, I was always picked last for the team. Most of the kids didn't want the fat kid that couldn't run or hit or shoot the ball on their team.

Moving on, I was always taught to finish my food or clean my plate. This was not a problem for me at the time, considering I was usually the first to finish my plate anyway. My Paw Paw always said, 'Take little bites,' and 'Chew your food slowly.' Mom would also say similar things, such as, 'No one's going to take your plate from you' and 'Slow down.'

I loved to eat. I would eat even when I wasn't hungry. Which leads me to believe I was an emotional eater when I was growing up. I was always encouraged to eat fruits and vegetables and good stuff like that, but most kids consider those types of food junk. If it isn't fried chicken or some fast food hamburger, I wasn't eating it. I did like bananas and apples, and I loved corn, too.

We never ate out very often when I was growing up. We mostly cooked at-home meals. When we did go out, it was almost always 'all you can eat' places, which was a big no-no with me. I could eat up to four or five plates if I ate at a buffet, mainly fried chicken and macaroni.

By the time I reached sixth grade, middle school, at the age of 14, I weighed 270 pounds. So from third grade to sixth grade, I gained almost 90 pounds. I lost my Paw Paw during that time. This resulted in some major emotional eating.

Around this time I started going to a family doctor. I believe I had the best doctor there is. He was always so kind and straight to the point. He watched me gain most of my weight. He tried to help me lose weight with the help of my parents. I mean, we tried almost everything. Diet pills, exercise, gyms, depression pills, thyroid pills, etc. We hadn't tried everything though. When I turned 17, my doctor informed me about the RNY surgery (gastric bypass surgery).

Most doctors will not perform the surgery on a 17-year-old. I had to wait a year to be eligible to have surgery, because of my age. I already had a fatty liver, high blood pressure (hypertension), and high cholesterol, and I had just found out I had sleep apnea, so I had to sleep with a mask to help me breathe at night.

When my 18th birthday came around, I weighed 468 pounds. I had gained almost 200 pounds in four years. My primary care doctor told me to go see a gastric bypass surgeon. The doctor said I was a very good candidate for surgery. I had to go through a six-month process of going to workshops on gastric bypass surgery and visiting a psychologist. I also had to see a nutritionist about my eating habits. She gave me a chart of what I should expect to eat after surgery and how much to eat at each meal. I had an overall evaluation with the psychologist to see if I was indeed ready for a major change to my lifestyle. She talked with the surgeon and let him know she did not think I was ready for surgery. 'What do I do now?' was going through my head when I got the news. I called my primary care physician and let him know about the evaluation. Without hesitation, he faxed a letter to both the psychologist and my surgeon, letting them know my life was at stake and that he was asking them to rethink the decision that was made.

After all this, I finally got the phone call stating that I could indeed go ahead with surgery. A date was set! 12-14-2009. Was I ready? Would it work? Would I make it out of the surgery alive? All these thoughts were running through my head. I got my head straight and was now ready to do this . . . or was I?

The day the surgery came around, I had to be at the hospital at 6:30 a.m. I got up and got ready for my big day. With my family surrounding me, I was now ready to go through with this life-changing journey.

I had my first doctor's visit after surgery and had lost about 30 pounds in the first three weeks. After my first six weeks I had lost about 50 to 60 pounds.

I was told at my next doctor's visit about the support group. It is an awesome group. Whenever you lose weight, up to 25 pounds and so on, you get a star with your weight loss on it. I love this.

With the support of family and friends, along with the support group and my awesome doctors, I am proud of how far I have come on this journey. I am almost two years out and have lost a total of 262 pounds and am now in size 32 pants. I started at a size 48. I'm in a large shirt, but had worn an XXXXL. Not to forget the most important part—and my whole reason for doing the surgery: I no longer have a fatty liver, high blood pressure, high cholesterol, or sleep apnea. I have done what so many overweight people dream of, which is 'being healthy'.

I truly believe that if I hadn't had the gastric bypass surgery, I would be dead by now. It's safe to say that gastric bypass has changed my life for the best. I'm not done with this, and I don't have a goal weight, because many people stop at their goal and say, 'I'm done.' The truth is—obesity is an addiction that we will all be struggling with for the rest of our lives."

I have a confession to make. I was the psychologist who suggested this young man was not ready for weight loss surgery at the time of his evaluation. I was not against his having weight loss surgery—I am never against that! For a number of reasons, I simply wanted him to demonstrate some specific healthy behaviors for a period of time prior to having the surgery. I am so proud for him that he has become such a great example to other young people in our community, as well as to all of those in the active WLS community where we live. He and I have talked at length about the reasons I had for wanting him to wait a bit and to implement some healthy behavior before having his surgery. We take advantage of our interaction when we are at support group meetings and use his situation as an example for others. He is very motivating and a wonderful young man!

Another male contributor, who spent years of his life in near social isolation, shared how his weight loss surgery has led to a much richer life:

"I moved to a new school in the middle of second grade, and by fourth grade was active in sports. It was baseball in the spring, soccer in the summer, football in the fall, and basketball in the winter. I enjoyed it, and was pretty good in baseball . . . and, from what I remember—not too bad at the other sports. I was also involved with Cub Scouts and later Boy Scouts. I loved the camping and such.

I didn't have a dad at home, though. My parents divorced when I was around three because my dad was an alcoholic. By about fourth grade, my mom had a boyfriend (they married a couple years later), but he was a drug user. Marijuana. I didn't know much about it at the time. I was aware of it, and I knew it was 'wrong,' but never really thought there was anything I could or should do about it.

Throughout elementary school I had 'friends'; I was active in doing things, but I also remember never feeling like I was really 'part of the gang.' I think later in life I wanted to believe it was because I was the 'fat kid,' but in looking back at photos from that time, I really wasn't fat. I might have been a bit taller than average, but I wasn't overweight. I guess by letting myself think it was because of my weight, I didn't have to consider what else it might have been . . . and its possible role in why I did gain weight.

The photos don't really show it as I remember, but I have memories of going to Weight Watchers meetings with my mom when I was in fifth grade. I've since asked her about it, but she doesn't recall it, so I don't know why I started going . . . or what, if anything, really came of it.

We moved after seventh grade, so I started a new school for eighth grade. The weight gain must have started by this point because I remember gym class. At that time the schools supplied uniforms, which were shirts and shorts. I had one of the largest shirts they had, and I remember the uncomfortable tightness of it around my gut. Oh, the anxiety I felt knowing the shirt just didn't fit. I remember a couple of times when other students referred to me as 'Porky . . .' followed by my last name, which also starts with 'Por.'

By eleventh grade, I was back at Weight Watchers. I remember losing weight, and using that as a justification to have various treats when I was at school. Peanut-butter Rice Krispie bars with chocolate on top were among my favorites.

Other than the few instances in eighth grade, I don't remember any real teasing about my weight. But I think it very much put me into a shell for about the next year. I don't remember much about ninth grade other than going to school and coming home. I started trying to venture out of my shell in tenth grade . . . playing football in the fall and then getting involved in the drama department (stage crew) after that, and I started making a few good friends, but overall I was still very much a loner. I had groups that I was on the fringes of, and in some ways very much a part of, but I still felt like an outsider, like I didn't really fit in.

I had felt this way when I was younger, and it only seemed to intensify as I got older. I think a lot of it was a result of the drug use by my stepfather. He wasn't just using, though, he was also selling it from our house. Even though we had a nice house with a big yard and a game room that included darts, pinball, and a pool table, I had no desire to try and invite people over in case they would find out about the drugs.

I had a couple of friends who lived on the same block as me who knew about the drugs, but when we did things, it was rarely at my house. We never actually talked about the situation. It wasn't until near the end of my senior year that I told my best friend at the time about it.

So yes, I had a few friends in high school, but I was always very awkward socially. I was the proverbial wallflower. I was afraid to ask girls out, and the only dance I attended in all of high school was Senior Prom, which I went to with a friend. Okay, I had a couple of 'girl friends' in high school, but I had no clue what I was doing . . . what it was about. Looking back, I realize it was the start of a very bad pattern when it came to my relationships with women.

There were many times I felt a lot of outright hatred for my stepfather. But even as young as 13 or 14, I knew I wouldn't have to live with it forever. My mom was happy (at least as far as I knew at the time), so I could put up with it. Yet I knew it would only be a matter of time before I could leave. So for her happiness, I put up with it.

Mom wasn't around for meals much, since she worked nights as a waitress and bartender. For whatever reason (likely the drugs, but I don't know for sure), my stepfather didn't keep steady employment. So I know my mom worked like heck to keep a roof over our heads and all that. Meals were often your basic 'meat and potatoes,' because that's what the stepdad liked. Usually something mom could fix ahead of time or easy things like burgers and fries that he could cook. As we got older (I have a sister who's 18 months younger), we would sometimes be responsible for cooking dinner. I enjoyed cooking, and would sometimes take the opportunity to try different things.

Overall, however, healthy eating was not something that was thought about in our house. I know my mom 'struggled' with weight all my life. While she doesn't really remember me going to Weight Watchers with her, it was something that was almost a constant for her over the years. Even with her working on her feet all the time . . . to this day . . . her weight is a struggle for her. But it's not something either of us remembers talking about. I don't know whose idea it was for me to go to Weight Watchers. I don't remember any comments from the stepfather (who was rail thin no matter what he ate). But it wouldn't surprise me to find out we never talked about such things. I know my mom's mom was that way—very repressed when it came to expressing feelings. Grandma died when I was in high school, but I don't know if I even remember ever giving her a hug or anything like that.

Then again, looking back, I'm sometimes surprised by how little I actually remember. I can't help but wonder if it's normal . . . or maybe it's just that I don't want to remember. Was it as bad as I think, or is it just the tendency to remember the bad more than the good?

At the same time, however, there are those same feelings that I continue to struggle with to this day. The feelings of still being on the outside. The social isolation. The anxiety. It's gotten better, by leaps and bounds . . . but it's still there.

Throughout my twenties I worked in restaurants, so I was on my feet all the time, and that helped keep me somewhat active, but my weight crept upwards. I had a small circle of friends—

very small. I was dating a woman, and was roommates with my best friend from high school along with her boyfriend. That was my circle. Both of those relationships ended, and my social interaction was limited to talking with co-workers and customers while at work and with people I was meeting online.

This was the early years of America Online, and I had more 'friends' from around the country than I did around where I lived. It was so much easier to talk—to approach someone—when they couldn't see you, couldn't judge you based on how much you weighed. It went on like this for a number of years. I didn't go out and do things. I stayed in and chatted with people from my computer. I suppose this only helped cement some of the bad eating habits I had. And my weight continued to creep upward. By the time I was 30, I probably weighed over 300 pounds.

Eventually though, I started chatting with folks from my area, not just across the country. It led to my meeting people face to face through organized group events. And some of those folks are my dearest friends to this day. It even led to a few relationships here and there, but that early pattern had been set up, and I was stuck in it. There were plenty of women I was attracted to, but would never dare to approach and ask out. I was 'the friend,' the 'nice guy' they would come to for a shoulder to cry on. As much as I secretly wished for more, I guess I was okay with that, thinking it was the best I could do. I had been in a couple of other relationships and they never lasted. I wasn't with them because of how I felt for them, but rather because of how I thought they felt for me. And I figured it was the best I was going to do.

Over the years, I had tried a couple of diets here and there. I would lose 20, 30, or even 40 pounds. But the loss would stall. I would get frustrated, and I would return to my old eating habits and the pounds would return . . . with friends.

By the time I was 33 or 34 I had resigned myself to two things: 1) that my weight was what it was, and 2) that I would be alone. I would be that old guy, sitting on the front steps by myself, wearing Bermuda shorts and sandals with black socks, watering the grass with the hose and threatening to spray any kids that got too close to my lawn.

During this time, it's not like I wasn't 'active.' Because of my muscle mass, nobody believed I weighed over 300 pounds (I was probably 340-ish at this point). I camped and hiked; I could easily hike 5 to 10 miles in a day. I had been playing sand-volleyball with a bar-league group, and at this point I had started playing paintball on a regular basis. Others were always amazed at how I could find cover behind trees much smaller than I was. I had to—there weren't that many trees that could fully cover me. So yeah, I wasn't exactly an athlete, but I was fairly active.

I was involved in other things too, like a living history educational group. Through the earlier group events with the AOL folks and things like this, I was doing okay talking to folks in groups. One-on-one, however, I was still pretty much shut down, and still very much a wallflower. I think it's because it's much easier not showing too much of yourself in a group situation.

Then I met 'her.' The first woman in my life I could say I actively pursued. I don't know what it was about her, but I was attracted to her almost from the first time I laid eyes on her. Over the summer, we became closer and closer and even intimate. My lack of experience in relationships kept me from being able to recognize how messed up things were. When we were alone, it was like we were a couple. When we were around others, we were just friends. When we were alone, we were intimate. When around others, I couldn't even hold her hand.

I convinced myself that she just needed time. She had recently been in a very serious relationship and just wasn't ready to acknowledge getting into another. I would try to give her space, and she would do something to draw me closer. I felt wanted, I felt . . . loved. And I could actually say I felt the same about her. I was very conscious of my weight in the relationship. Part of me couldn't believe what was happening. She was actually the thinnest woman I had ever been in a relationship with, and she actually seemed to care about me, to want to be with me? There were days it was just mind-boggling for me.

Well, I wasn't wrong, but I wasn't entirely right either. I don't doubt that she loved me, that she wanted me, but it just wasn't in quite the same way that I loved her, that I wanted her. Suddenly, before I really knew what had happened, she was dating someone else, publicly. None of the 'only when alone' sort of stuff we had. To make matters worse, at least in my mind, he was not even half my size. He was 'normal.' To say I was devastated would be an understatement. I fell into a serious depression. I wasn't sleeping. I wasn't eating. In a matter of months I lost nearly 50 pounds and got the closest I had been to getting under 300 for the first time in seven or eight years.

Slowly I came out of it. But as my life started returning to normal, so did the pounds. And they came back with a vengeance. Soon I was back over 350 pounds, and then some.

I mentioned paintball. This was still my favorite form of recreation. But as I shot past 350 pounds and then 360, getting around on the field was getting harder and harder. Hiking, something I loved doing when camping, didn't seem like much of an option when just walking out to get the mail made my lower back hurt. And forget about getting down on the floor to play with my niece and nephew.

We had a paintball team, a group of us that played on a regular basis. And while getting out to the field and playing was a struggle for me, to the point I wasn't really playing much, I still wanted to be a part of things. So instead, I would go out on the field with a camera to take photos of others playing. One of those players was Larry. Larry had turned 60 shortly after I first met him, and here it was a few years later and he was still out on that field. Had I tried to run, he would have run circles around me.

People ask what my 'aha' moment was, the moment I decided to have weight loss surgery. There wasn't a single moment, but a culmination of some small things. Between not playing paintball, not being able to play with my niece and nephew, not being able to walk without back pain, and looking at my friend Larry, I finally realized that if I didn't do something, not only would I never be like Larry, out there playing paintball 20 years in the future, I likely wouldn't be here at all.

This was the fall of 2008. My aunt, who had been morbidly obese all my life, had RNY earlier in the year and was having some good success with it. Before that, I had always told myself I should be able to lose weight on my own. I knew what I needed to do. Eat better, eat less, and exercise. It's so simple. But it was never easy. I finally realized I couldn't do it alone. I needed help.

I attended my first appointment at the surgeon's office in October. Just before Thanksgiving, I was put on the pre-op weight loss plan by the nutritionist. My goal was to lose 21 pounds (for shrinking the liver and such) before surgery. I stuck with the 1,500-calorie-a-day plan they put me on, and by New Year's I was down nearly 30 pounds.

I started having second thoughts. This was going so much easier than it had ever seemed to before. And yet . . . there was always that 'before' to consider. I'd been down this road too many times. Plus, although I wouldn't say that during the pre-op dieting stage I was 'always hungry,' I also knew I was 'never full.' I realized surgery would give me that help I needed in that regard. So I pushed on, and by the time I was approved and in the hospital waiting for my surgery in April of 2009, I was down nearly 60 pounds from my heaviest (which was somewhere over 380, but I was never weighed at my heaviest point).

The nearly three years since I had my surgery have been kind of a blur. At about six months out, I weighed under 230 pounds, having lost nearly 100 pounds since surgery. I was smaller than I was when I graduated high school. I started considering dating and tried some online sites. I met some nice women, and went out a few times, but soon realized I wasn't ready. My head was still very much playing catch-up.

I became very active in the weight loss surgery community: blogging, doing videos, volunteering at my surgeon's office to speak to others considering surgery, and more. And I was playing again. Playing with my niece and nephew. I was their favorite jungle gym. Playing paintball, more than ever and moving around the field like I never had before. Just before surgery I bought a bike, a hulk of a mountain bike, because I was still over 320 pounds. At that point I would have been happy to hit 250, and I figured I would need a bike to stand up to my weight.

The first time I rode (I tried once just before surgery), I could barely go a mile before I got wiped out. By the end of that summer, I was doing 10-mile treks on that bike. The summer of 2010, I put 700 miles on my bike, including a trip to see my mom one Sunday. She lives 20 miles from me.

It's cliché, but here I was, in my early forties, feeling better than I had in my early thirties or even late twenties. At about 16 months post-op, I tried the dating thing again. I met a wonderful woman, and we started dating pretty seriously, pretty quickly, actually. During this time I got laid off, and with her encouragement I turned it into an opportunity to pursue a whole new career path in nutrition.

Unfortunately, the relationship didn't last. As much as I've changed, and after everything I've done these last few years, there are still things from my past I have yet to overcome. Relationships are one of those things I am still working on. I don't know if it's because of issues related to my parents and stepdad, or just because of those years of social isolation, but there are many things about being in a relationship I'm just not very good at.

In a lot of ways, post-op life is a sort of a 'do-over.' I am getting a chance to do things I never could have, never would have imagined when I was living inside a 350-pound body. Physically, mentally, and emotionally. Even though the weight loss was rapid, thanks to the RNY, dealing with the changes it brings is something that takes time.

When asked about surgery and if they have any regrets, a lot of people like to say 'my only regret is not having done this sooner.' I can't say that. I wish I had, but I also know I wasn't ready. I wasn't at a point where I would have been able to make the commitment it takes to make this work. Again—physically, mentally, and emotionally. But thanks to that decision to have the surgery, I know I have the time."

This risk-taking man did not let the shame of his stepfather's use and selling of marijuana from the family home, or the shame related to his weight, interfere with his making and maintaining contact with others outside the home. He continued to seek companionship with others even though he felt intimidated. He was living a recovery slogan before he began his recovery from obesity! "Feel the fear and do it anyway!" is one of the most powerful recovery slogans. Of course he felt fear—he had never been in the "inner circle" of a group, where every teenager wants to be. He continued to reach out, if only online, for people with whom he felt secure. Although he did not obtain a true sense of security with most of the people with whom he interacted until recent years, he continued to reach out to them and maintain some level of interaction. He took charge of getting his needs met, rather than waiting for other people in his life to change or waiting for others to meet his needs for him. This man behaved in a way that reflects "adult thinking" versus "child thinking" as described by John Friel, PhD:

Child Thinking	Adult Thinking
I'm trapped.	I'm accountable.
I wait for others to make my life better.	I have choices.
I wait for others to change.	I find appropriate ways to meet my needs.
I wait for others to give me what I deserve.	I take charge of what needs to happen. I can choose not to change, but then I don't blame others . . . or . . . I choose to change.

In his adult life, the contacts he made prior to his surgery are the people with whom he has developed healthy, adult in-person relationships. For many people, obesity is strongly related to a felt inability to have genuine, meaningful relationships. This man did not have a father with whom to relate or to teach him about how to have friendships with boys and later with men. He did not have a mother who was around enough to give him individual attention. Neither his father nor his stepfather taught him to have a healthy relationship with a female. This contributor has had to figure out a lot of things on his own. By his own admission, he continues to work through many of his questions and seeks to find answers. He has grown tremendously as a person and in his relationships as his body has shrunk following weight loss surgery three years ago!

Take a good look at the "child thinking" versus "adult thinking" chart above. Make a copy of it and post it in several areas where you will see it often: at your office, in your bedroom, on the bathroom mirror, and hey—make a laminated mini-copy to carry in your wallet. Whether you're dealing with a food decision, an internal battle about whether or not to exercise, or how to handle a situation with a co-worker, a spouse, or a sibling, use the chart and remember that you are an adult. The truth is that most of us were not taught to respond like adults in a lot of situations, but were taught by our role models to react using childlike thinking when dealing with people and situations in our lives. Use those same trailblazing skills you are using to develop a life of healthy eating and exercise behaviors to implement healthy adult communication skills with those in your family and social life as well! The bottom line: we are each responsible for recognizing our needs and getting them met in healthy ways (which means no blaming others, waiting for them to change, or to give me what I "deserve").

The above paragraph is an example of one of my tangents. Hey, I have to seize the moment! And since I'm on Tangent Trail, I'll throw in one more thought. About obesity and relationships. Relationships, as noted by the contributor above, are affected by obesity. For good or bad, there are people who would not consider having a relationship with an obese person. I'm not judging this as being right or wrong; I'm simply stating it as being a reality—for some people. Similarly, there are people who wouldn't consider having a relationship with a redhead or a bald person or a woman with short hair. People have preferences. For an obese person, however, this can be a painful and frustrating matter related to their weight and relationships. One they have no control over (as in—we can't control another person's relationship preferences).

The obese person also has an impact on the quality of his or her own relationships. Depending on the self-esteem of the obese person, interpersonal relationships can be severely negatively impacted. If people have a regular commentary of negative self-talk flowing through their brains, reminding them how "horrible" or "worthless" or "unworthy" or "undeserving" or "stupid" or "ugly" or "out of control" or "fat" they are, my guess is they are not going to be all that pleasant to be around. Remember, thoughts affect our feelings and our attitudes and our behaviors. While we might smile pretty and act nice to the people at work all day, we may go home and take our personal unhappiness out on our partners and children.

Obesity is a family disease. Nearly all interpersonal relationships are affected by a person's obesity. Children often act as "gophers" for the obese person—going for this or going for that because the obese parent is too tired or physically unable to get up and move around comfortably. Spouses may work diligently to try to make things as easy as possible for the obese partner, and may be overwhelmed by needing to take on the majority of responsibilities. Perhaps they are silently resentful of doing the extra caretaking of children, preparation of meals, and going to doctor's appointments. Maybe the spouse is upset about the lack of an intimate relationship as a result of their partner's obesity.

Following significant weight loss, relationships change. In many ways, for the better. Families are able to participate in activities they could not do together before the surgery. The parent who lost weight is able to attend kids' activities and spouse's company events. Sexual relationships may resume in a marriage. All members of the family may begin to eat healthier foods and participate in more exercise. In many ways, one person's weight loss can have a positive impact on everyone in the family.

If you are the person who has lost the weight, please watch carefully for any signs by your spouse or your kids that may suggest they may be displeased in some ways after you lose weight. It's usually not that they are unhappy about the weight loss. It's about the ways your relationship with them changes. For example, what about that child who was your personal "gopher?" If you are now able to get your own things, the child may feel he has lost his "role" in your life. It's not that the kid wants to have to fetch things for you, it's that he wants to be important to you. Help him feel important in new ways—by helping you plan a menu or cooking with you. Have him participate in choosing family activities.

Every week I hear someone say, "My spouse makes jokes that I won't want him (or her) now that I've lost weight." We all know that is not a joke. When one spouse or partner loses weight, that often leads to improved self-esteem, better boundary-setting and a busier social life, and the spouse or partner may feel insecure about the relationship. I promise you these personal improvements are going to result in changes in relationships.

The couples and families who talk about these things openly and directly, sharing their thoughts and feelings, will get through the process so much more quickly and with fewer battle scars! Remember what I noted a few paragraphs ago—few of us learned about healthy communication skills from our adult role models. That makes it difficult to know how to have conversations about feeling vulnerable "because I worry that you won't want or need me not that you've lost weight and are looking great and doing so much more than you used to. . . ."

Be sensitive to the needs of your loved ones. Kids don't have the skills to articulate their thoughts and feelings unless they have been taught how. Spouses don't either. So if you find that all of a sudden there seem to be more problems in the relationships at home than there were before you lost weight, get some help from a professional who can guide everyone through it. Changes are difficult on everyone involved. Having someone help you verbalize what you're thinking and feeling helps you realize that what you are going through is normal and can help you talk with one another. Your family members need reassurance that you still love, want, and need them, even though you are now many pounds lighter.

One last thing—I promise! Sure, self-esteem usually improves as you lose weight, but the habit of negative self-talk doesn't automatically go away, and self-esteem improvements that last (i.e., don't fluctuate in direct proportion to changes on the scale on any given day) don't usually happen solely due to weight loss. The bottom line: your issues remain largely the same before and after weight loss. Until you deal with whatever the underlying issues are, they will affect your relationships, regardless of your weight. *So*, as I always suggest, "Get help and get happy!"

Now, back to the original topic. The following paragraphs are responses by a variety of contributors who were overweight or obese in childhood. They share what it was like for them to go through such an important stage of life being heavy:

"I was very overweight as a child, but I did not let it stop me from having friends and living my life. As I reached puberty, life became more difficult for me. My peers were dating and going out, and I was staying home and feeling self-conscious. I focused on my studies. I was on diets as a child. My mother was always watching her weight and she was concerned about my weight problem. Doctors could not find anything wrong with me. Mom was careful about monitoring my food intake and kept no fattening food in the house. This continued throughout my life, into adulthood."

"I was teased more by my family than by friends. My grandmother had suggestions on how I should eat, like to only have open-faced sandwiches. I think that was my first 'diet' that I remember. I was always made to feel inferior to my younger, slimmer sister. She was smarter, skinnier, and prettier my whole life. She was gorgeous—all the boys said so. They said I was cute. I did go out for track but I was nowhere near as good at it as my sister was. I didn't hang out with the girls because they were judgmental. The boys were my friends, I had no girl friends. I was chunky when I lived with my grandmother because she wasn't watching the fridge and I could sneak in there and eat whatever was there."

"I was a very heavy child and yes, always teased. I was able to stand up for myself, although I retaliated in different ways to express my anger about it. I was extremely unhappy and hated myself. I tried to gain attention because I thought no one cared about me. I absolutely hated any form of exercise, especially at school, but because the teacher knew that, she forced me to participate even more so. I remember pretending to break my hand one time. I put on a bandage, but she then caught me in cooking class without it!"

"'So-Fat.' . . . Those two words still haunt me. I can't remember ever being thin, so obesity has just been part of my life. To my dad and sisters my nickname was 'Fatso' as far back as I can remember. One day in my early teens I remember my dad saying that 'Fatso' didn't make sense, so they were going to start calling me 'So-Fat.' From that day forward I was 'So-Fat' to members of my immediate family. To this day I can't shake those memories. In my school days I had a few close friends, but tended to be a loner and didn't participate in any sports or activities. I remember many times going to school on Monday only to hear about all of the fun activities that my 'friends' did over the weekend. I am not sure if it's true, but I always felt like they didn't invite me because I was fat and they were embarrassed to be my friend."

As I read these words that describe the actual experiences of real human beings, my heart aches. I want to pretend and believe that these are stories written to teach people what it would be like for children to be picked on by others. But these are the actual lives of human beings who were children at one time.

Does it make sense to you for even a minute that these children would not have permanent scars on their hearts and in their minds as a result of this type of treatment? Note that I said "permanent scars." Meaning that simply adding years to their lives doesn't make the pain of those experiences go away. Although the wounds aren't seen as gaping, bleeding sores—wow, as I write this, I am trying to imagine what it would look like if the pain of emotional hurts were visible and looked like the wounds caused by a rock that hits someone's head or a tree branch that was scraped down an arm or a sharp object drug across one's heart. We wouldn't ignore children walking around with those visible sorts of wounds. And hopefully, we would all be a whole lot more careful about inflicting them if we could literally see what damage we were causing. Trust me, the scars left from those emotional wounds are on the hearts, in the minds, and deep in the souls of all children teased, bullied, and called names about their weight. As you read more from the courageous contributors to this book, try to imagine what they would have looked like if their hurts had been visible to everyone they passed by:

"I was overweight as a child. Not severely, but I was very self-conscious about this. I felt like I was the odd one out when everyone was thinner. It was horrible at gym class when everyone was weighed. Specifically in sixth grade. Most everyone was 98 pounds; I was 126. Of course the weights were called out by the gym teacher, and I was humiliated. I was teased by friends who called me 'Fat Fingers.' It doesn't sound so bad now at age 50, but at age 8 it was horrible."

"I was heavy as a child, big for my age. I really don't remember being teased by my friends or by the kids at school. My issues with my weight were really basically from family. One of the painful memories I have is of my grandmother comparing my thighs to her waist when I was about 10 years old. This is where all the pain about my weight as a child really stems from.
My mother had/has her own body issues, and she projected those issues on me. She put me on every diet she went on and gave me every pill she took for herself. This included having my pediatrician prescribe amphetamines for me when I was about 10 years old. Can you imagine giving a 10-year-old speed? In the third grade she would take me to this one particular diet doctor three days a week before school to get shots. That was such a wonderful way to start the day for a child terrified of needles. She would drag me in there kicking and screaming and crying . . . but it never made a difference. I remember one diet in particular that I hated. It required me eating half [of] a grapefruit before every meal, and every meal consisting of spinach and boiled eggs along with some kind of meat. I never really thought about being heavy as a child except in context with what my mother was doing to me, and when someone would say something to me. I was not allowed to leave the house if there was not an adult home, so I would often watch TV and eat. If there was an adult home, I would be outside riding my bike or traveling all over the neighborhood. We would play hide-and-seek using the whole

block. Yes, I had friends. In fact, I am still friends with someone I met when I was six years old from the neighborhood we lived in at the time.

I was and I wasn't a loner. At school I think I was more of a loner. I was shy, but not when I got to know someone. When I was very young, my mother's boss paid for me to take dance lessons with her daughters who were my age. I have a vague memory of that, and I remember doing the Brownie thing.

I don't remember my weight being a hindrance to anything I wanted to do—at least not so that I was aware of it. I don't remember avoiding anything because of my weight. I would exclude myself from any activity where my mother was involved. I would go hide in my bedroom, read, and eat. Looking back at pictures of myself, I don't really think that I was that heavy. But it became a kind of a self-fulfilling prophecy. I was always being told how fat I was by my mother and being made to feel as if I was not good enough because of the way I looked."

"I didn't really have a weight problem until high school. However, I did blossom early, so I was teased some about that. And ever since I was very little, my dad called me 'Porky.' He called me that for years, and it bothered me.

My parents were divorced when I was about eight, and I was forced to live with my dad. My mom was obese, and my dad would always tell me to stop acting like my mom. Oh, I hated it. That is when the self-esteem issues began, I think.

By the time I got to high school, I was overweight, but not huge. I did get teased, and of course I didn't like it. It kept me from doing things like swimming because there was no way I'd wear a suit. I shied away from many things throughout high school, and for me . . . high school was quite miserable.

My dad dealt drugs and during the summer between my eighth- and ninth-grade years, I turned him in so I could have a chance to live with Mom.

Living with Mom is when my weight began to go up. She would work a long week and figured on the weekend we deserved to go to dinner. It was generally a buffet place. Mom wasn't active, either. Her lazy lifestyle was easy to pick up. Because I didn't have transportation and was too shy anyway, I was never involved with after-school activities. I had a few friends, but not many.

My grandparents were always concerned about weight, but
my mom didn't listen. I was young and didn't give it a whole lot
of thought. Looking back, I don't think I was terribly overweight
in high school at all. I just thought I was. I definitely wasn't the little size 6. I was more like a size 12 with more of an athletic build.
But all I saw was fat and ugly. I constantly dogged on myself and
led myself to believe that that is what I was."

In recent years, one of the ways teens, in particular, have
attempted to deal with their inner, emotional pain is to cause physical damage to their bodies via cutting themselves. People are mortified when they hear about this, wondering how in the world anyone
could do such harm to themselves. If you talk to people who cut
themselves, they will tell you that cutting and the resulting physical
pain is so much less intense than the hurt they feel on the inside.

How different is the cutter from the bulimic or the people who
gorge themselves to the point of physical fullness so that they can
barely move? How different is cutting oneself from the "dogging
on myself" the previous contributor noted? Many of the people
who wrote for this book note how they began to hate themselves
and say horrible things to themselves. That's what children do
when they are bullied, teased, constantly criticized, expected to be
perfect, and called derogatory names. They start doing it to themselves. How aware are you that you may still be "dogging" yourself
as an adult? Recognizing your negative self-talk and negative treatment of yourself is imperative so you can change it and the ways
you feel about yourself!

The messages people get about food and eating also have a
lasting impact in terms of how we make food choices as adults.
Contributors discussed what messages they learned at home about
eating and about food:

"If I were still hungry after a meal, my mother would not allow
me another helping of food. She would tell me the hunger was in
my head. She told me what to eat and what not to eat. Once I was

living on my own, I started eating the foods I wanted and gained more weight. I finally felt free from the restrictions at home."

"I was encouraged to eat differently than the other kids. Somehow I didn't get the impression that I was the same as them or had the same value. I was given a jar of homemade pickled watermelon rinds by my maternal grandmother and I snuck to the refrigerator over and over until the whole jar was gone the afternoon I opened it. My grandmother didn't leave her chair during the day after she'd been drinking and it was easy to do."

"My mom was an emotional eater, and I became an emotional eater. My mom and her husband were both morbidly obese. They worked during the day. I had the school hot lunch, which was usually some burger equivalent to a Big Mac, or pizza. There weren't many healthy options. After school we'd come home and have some sort of snack—whatever we could find because no parents were around. Then we'd have dinner, and that could've been anything. A lot of times there was ice cream before bed. The diet wasn't the healthiest. Because my mom was overweight, she didn't say a whole lot to me about it. She always told me I wasn't fat and that I looked fine. Oh yes, we were taught to clean our plates. Food was a part of every celebration too. When I would visit my dad, he never said anything about eating healthy or exercising—he would just always tease me about being fat. No advice, nothing. He was an emotional abuser, in my opinion. Between my dad teasing me and my mom having poor eating habits and a lazy lifestyle, I was headed toward obesity."

"My father died when I was seven. Mother had to work to support three growing sons. I ate what was put on the table, so I learned to eat a lot of stuff most kids would not eat. I was left to fix my own breakfast, so toast and peanut butter was it most of the time."

"I love my parents so much, but my mom will admit she hates to cook. She would make things like casseroles and TV dinners. With both of my parents being in education, we would eat most meals at the dinner table together. I miss that. We would go out to eat at least once a week for either Friday night fish fry or

Hardee's. We would go out to eat at a nice restaurant very few times a year and usually considered it a treat. I ended up treating myself almost every day as an adult.

We were expected to eat everything on our plates. My brother hated vegetables, so I would usually help him eat those, especially squash. Yummy. Foods such as candy bars, potato chips, and Ding Dongs were always a treat. They were never readily available at home. When I was trying to raise money for German club to go to Germany, we were selling candy bars. I ate more bars than I sold and then had to put forward the money. My entire allowances were going towards my sugar bingeing. I also remember when I was a junior in high school, I began to eat two lunches at school. I would have my best friend walk through the line and get a lunch, even though she brought her own, just to get me an extra. I ate, and ate some more."

"I was allowed to eat anything I wanted; in fact, my mother always made sure I was fed and never ever told me I was fat. She would force me to eat everything on my plate because 'there were children starving in the world.' I loved it at the time, but thinking back now, I wish she had helped me with my obesity. She loved me unconditionally, I guess, and didn't want to hurt my feelings, but in the long run I totally suffered from it. Food was always an example of love in my house and a 'reward.'"

What a variety of experiences! Some people were told exactly what to eat and when to eat it. Some had very little supervision in regard to their food intake, even as children. This makes me think about something I speak of on a regular basis to groups of people when we get to the topic of parenting. One of the descriptions of the various forms of parenting I like best refers to three types of parents:

Authoritarian Parents:
- try to control their kids' behaviors and their attitudes, using a "this is the way it's always been done" mentality
- often have extremely strict rules, again in an attempt to control their children by being the "boss," and they often do so with a lack of affection and warmth

- tell children what to do, try to force compliance, and don't give kids choices or explanations for their decisions or behaviors
- focus on bad behavior, rather than positive behavior
- use harsh punishment, often including physical discipline
- "*my way or the highway*"

The Kids of Authoritarian Parents:

- have trouble learning to think and make decisions for themselves
- sometimes have trouble with social skills and interacting with other children
- struggle to take initiative
- become "bullies" themselves in response to being bullied by demanding parents who are often unresponsive to the children
- are often well-behaved (due to fear of punishment)
- lack resourcefulness, as they have always been told what to do and therefore haven't learned how to solve their own problems
- struggle with low self-esteem
- may do poorly in school
- often "act out" (they are acting out feelings they do not have the skills to verbalize, and they have no one with whom to discuss their feelings)

  If you had authoritarian parents, how might that have affected your eating?

Permissive Parents:

- give their kids a lot of freedom over their lives, including schedules, friends, and activities

- have minimal expectations about achievement and mature behavior from their children compared with other types of parents
- give kids too much input into decisions for selves and/or family
- do not exercise explicit control over their kids' behavior
  - ᐧ may believe kids need to learn from experience
  - ᐧ may not put forth the effort or involvement in their children's lives

The Kids of Permissive Parents:

- are often immature
- have trouble controlling impulses (because they've had no boundaries)
- struggle to accept responsibility for their own behaviors
- act independently

If you had permissive parents, how might that have affected your eating?

Authoritative Parents:

- recognize and accept that they are the parents and have more information and skills to make decisions than their children, but allow the children to have input and respect that they, too, have rights as people (to be heard, listened to, and taken into consideration)
- focus on obedience and respect for authority rather than using physical force to teach positive behaviors to children
- explain rules and decisions, allow input from children, but reserve the right as the parent to make the rules
- consider their children's points of view, while retaining the authority as the parent to make the final decisions
- encourage children to learn to make decisions, encourage them to be individuals and to be independent

- set goals and standards for their kids, providing rewards and consequences along with explanations
- Are *"firm and fair"*

The Kids of Authoritative Parents:
- are willing to explore and take risks as they have learned to be part of the decision-making process
- are respectful of family, parents, friends and, others
- are more self-confident and willing to risk and "fail," as it doesn't mean they are a "failure" and they have confidence based on approval and acceptance from parents
- are more emotionally stable
- feel more freedom to express themselves and their opinions and to state their needs due to being given consideration by their family members

If you had authoritative parents, how might that have affected your eating?

As you read some more comments from contributors about what they learned from their parents about food and eating, try to see if you can imagine what kind of parents they had!

"Eating healthy was not part of our family vocabulary. My mom didn't prepare meals, so we all just fended for ourselves. There were always plenty of frozen dinners or frozen pizza to microwave when we were hungry. If not, a bowl or two of cereal made a good supper.

LOL . . . talk about mixed messages. My mother put me on diets and diet pills, but then would keep all kinds of things like soda and cookies and chips in the house. There was always some kind of snack food there.

My little sister was the perfect one because she was naturally thin. . . . I don't know how I managed to keep from feeling jealous of her, but I never did. She was five years younger and was my mother's favorite. I knew that but never blamed my sister.

Knowing people and kids, it still amazes me that I was never jealous of her. I was always proud of her, actually.

The clean plate club is part of the mixed messages I had to deal with. My mother put me on diet pills, and my father would insist that I eat everything that was on my plate. I remember when she first started me on the diet pills (amphetamines) she measured out a half cup of peas and whatever else was on my plate. Do you have any idea how much a half a cup of peas is? It is a lot. There was no way I could eat what was on my plate, no way. I was taking speed! I remember looking at the food that was on that plate and bursting out in tears because they were going to make me eat what was there. I just couldn't do it. My father was yelling at me, and I was crying. He told me I had to sit there until I ate everything on my plate. So here I was, about 10 years old, on speed, having to sit at the table and stare at what looked like a huge plate of food, and I was not going to be allowed to leave the table until I cleaned my plate. The funny part of all of that is, had my mother not actually measured out the food, she would have put a lot less on my plate to begin with. I still would not have been able to eat it, but I think it would have been less traumatizing to me. To this day the only thing I remember are those peas. And I actually liked peas.

Again this was where the mixed messages came in. Food was the enemy on one hand, and the way we celebrated, on the other. We were always having people over for dinner. In the summertime it was great. We would cook out and make homemade ice cream. I remember snapping beans and shucking corn. We would go out on the boat, camp out on one of the islands in the river for the weekend, and no one would say anything to me about food. At other times, if I was good (or they just wanted to get rid of me), they would give me money to go to the store to buy candy."

Respondents discussed the messages they received about themselves from their parents:

"My father loved me unconditionally, regardless of my weight. He thought I was beautiful. I felt love from both my parents; however, I felt like I failed my mother, due to my weight. I still feel like this, even as an adult. I often felt that if I could have lost weight that I would have been loved more. When I was 19, I went on a crash diet, and my mother gave me so much praise. When the weight came back, it was a different story."

"My parents expected a lot from me because I was the oldest. I took care of my mom from age 6 to age 10, and that was a giant responsibility. Some days I would worry about what was happening to my mom at home and get 'sick' at school so that I could go home and make sure she was all right. I also had to lie down with my brother or sister when they needed to nap. I cleaned the house and did all sorts of chores for my mom because she was unable to move from the couch. I bathed her or helped her bathe. I even helped her in the toilet. I had a lot of responsibility. They always said I had such a level head on my shoulders. I never wanted to let them down. I felt sad sometimes because I never felt I was good enough."

This particular comment made me realize how often children are not really allowed to be children. This isn't an obesity-specific issue. In the case of this contributor, the mother had a serious illness. She had not done anything wrong. She didn't force her child to be an adult prematurely. In this case, the circumstances required that the kids in the household assume additional responsibilities because their mother had a debilitating disease, one that she could not alter with healthier behaviors.

No one was at fault here, and there is no blame to be doled out. Just compassion for a family whose lives were interrupted by multiple sclerosis. The fact remains that the person writing this account lost important parts of childhood because of MS. The child, rather than being able to focus on her "job," which was school, was worried about her mother and wanted to get home to care for her. This child likely experienced fear on a regular basis and had a tremendous amount of stress for a little one.

Chronic stress literally causes alterations in brain development in young people. My hope is that this writer takes some time with a good friend or therapist and talks about how multiple sclerosis robbed her of what might have been a carefree childhood and grieves over the fact that her childhood was very different from her friends'. Hers is an example of a progressive disease, not an abusive or irresponsible parent, robbing her of her childhood. The effects are often the same, regardless of what "steals" the good parts of being a kid.

Obesity is also a chronic disease. Fortunately, the obese person usually can alter, to some degree, the severity of the disease by making lifestyle changes. Sadly, many people don't recognize that they struggle to make the lifestyle changes permanent because there are layers of emotional issues surrounding the obesity. Having an obese parent, one with another chronic disease, one suffering from chemical or behavioral addictions, one with a serious mental illness, as well as a thousand other things that can happen in life, often result in children "growing up too fast." If you are one of those people, please take some time and allow yourself to grieve over what you missed during your childhood. Take the time, feel the feelings, talk about them, and then choose to make each day of your adult life a good one.

"Oh my gosh . . . from my dad I got the message that I was just a fat girl who couldn't do any better than her mom. It still angers me to this day. I think my mom was unaware that I had a weight problem in high school because she was so overweight. Of course I appeared thin to her. Due to my dad's teasing all the time, I was pretty much convinced that I would be fat forever. I found that most of the time I was sad. I was never brave enough to tell my dad how he made me feel."

"I was unaware I had a problem during my childhood years. I quit college my first year, moved to Chicago, and lost about 35 pounds while I lived there. I was hungry, but always ate very well. I discovered ethnic foods such as sushi and Thai. I met a girl who had been in *Vogue* magazine, and we worked out together almost every night. I got down to 137 pounds, but with a boyfriend who constantly commented about weight, I always felt self-conscious. I left him, moved back to Wisconsin, and went back to college. I also gained weight pretty quickly as I stopped working out. I continued to gain after college, finally hitting my heaviest of 283.

I was loved and never put down, but I was very embarrassed about my weight, and ashamed and very angry. I needed to be loved because of this.

The constant teasing and insecurities eventually led to me becoming anorexic. I lost 60 pounds during the summer after my sophomore year. After starting my junior year of school, the kids started teasing me about being too thin and would bug me all the time because I never ate anything. It seemed like I couldn't win. So I would eat to please people and then vomit when I got the chance, thus becoming bulimic. I struggled with this eating disorder for over a year. I have always had an 'all or nothing' personality, so eventually I just gave up again and gained all the weight back plus several more pounds.

My family told me I was beautiful. If I wanted to exercise they encouraged it, they encouraged me to follow my dreams, that I could be and do whatever I put my mind to.

This is the one area I don't think they sent me mixed messages. I was constantly being told that I was stupid, and lazy; I always felt worthless. I never felt as if I was good enough for them. I was told that I would never amount to anything. As a child I never really thought about my weight outside of the context of my mother. She would embarrass me. She would make me feel ashamed, especially when shopping for clothes.

Let's return to the idea of the parenting types explained earlier. Perhaps you found it easy to identify what type of parents the contributors in this chapter had. Maybe it was pretty clear what kinds of parents you had. Let's go a step further. Ask yourself what kind of parent you are or were. Maybe your kids are grown and you have regrets about some of the things you did as a parent (like most of us do). Perhaps you wish you had fed them differently. Maybe you wish you had given them more chores—or fewer chores. Maybe you realize that a particular nickname you had for them was funny to you, but looking back, can see how it may have been painful for them.

We've talked about breaking the chains of obesity in families. You have begun to do that by losing weight and incorporating the Gotta Do 'Ems to keep that weight off. You can continue to do so with your kids/grandkids, whether they are grown or still in your care. In her book *Breaking Free from Emotional Eating,* Geneen Roth provides parents with a list of things they can do to help kids learn to be healthy and responsible with food choices.

Parents can:

- allow their kids to take responsibility for food: take kids to the grocery store and consult with them about shopping and cooking

- post a grocery list on the fridge . . . instilling in them the sense that their decisions and feelings about food are important enough to be considered and acted upon

- allow kids to decide on one or two dinners per day: enlist their help in preparing, cooking and cleaning up

- talk about nutrition, read books together, plan meals based on what you read

- do not use the dinner hour to argue grievances, arbitrate fights, discipline, or have emotional discussions

- encourage your kids to develop trust in their ability to care for themselves, respect for their health and bodies, and a relationship with you in which they feel you are guiding them and walking with them instead of judging them, preaching to them, and doubting their autonomy. But first you must pay close attention to your own fear about your body: if you don't believe that your body will tell you when and what to eat it's going to be difficult to encourage that belief in your child. To foster a healthy relationship between your child and his or her body and food, you must also begin working with yourself on the issues of trust, body image, and self-worth.

You can also break the chain of poor parenting behaviors that may have been passed through generations of your family that have nothing to do with food. (I know, here I go. . . .). You want your over-all life improved after losing weight, so I'm just throwing a thought or two in to help you do so in other areas of life!

One of the best things we can give our children is an acknowl-edgment and apology, when appropriate, for things we did that have hurt them. For example, let's say you come from a family who, for generations, has demonstrated anger by screaming and shouting and calling names. Your parents did it to you, and you turned out all right . . . right? (I threw that line in there because it drives me crazy. I always want to ask, "What do you mean when you say that you turned out all right?") You survived. We all survived if we're still alive. But did the screaming and hollering scare you when you were a kid? What did you learn to do to cope with the fear? Eat too much? Learn to keep your thoughts and feelings to yourself, hoping the hollering would end sooner? Did the name-calling hurt your feelings? Lead to your doubting yourself? Cause you to develop a habit of negative self-talk?

If you, as a parent, carried on the tradition of screaming and yelling and name-calling and are now realizing that you may have frightened your children or damaged their self-esteem when they were growing up—then tell them! Let them know you realize it may have been hard for them to listen to all that noise. Acknowl-edge it had to hurt their feelings when you would call them (or their siblings or other parent) names. Tell them you know it was wrong, that you are sorry, and that you apologize. What a gift you would be giving them. And just as importantly, you would be show-ing them how to apologize to their own children, and help them realize they can parent in healthier ways. And *that* is how healthy behaviors get passed on to new generations!

Erin Akey, the Bariatric Guru, writes an incredibly powerful blog, noting the ways you can, as you lose weight, change the patterns in your family's attitudes and behaviors toward health. In this blog, Erin directly shares the importance of including our families in the journey toward health following WLS. Erin (who sounds to me like a very healthy Authoritative parent), notes the responsibility we, as parents, have for helping our children transition into the healthier lifestyle, as they are not the ones who signed up for it when their parents made the decision to have WLS. Erin also makes it clear that, as the parents, we are responsible for what our children eat in our homes and where we take them out to eat. This is a great post entitled, "What are we doing to our kids????? And WHY????"

"I used to be morbidly obese. Most of you know that. I was 326 pounds in 2008 and had gastric bypass and decided to take control of my life and get my health back. I am a work in progress and will be forever. I was forced to face my food addiction and to completely change my life. Just like an alcoholic has to live with their addiction daily, so do I.

FACTS: These tend to be true for many of us who were once morbidly obese and who lost the weight. It does not matter if you lost your weight through surgical or non-surgical means, the facts are still likely to apply to you if you grew up as an obese child and young adult. If you are still obese, then you can really relate to these, I am sure.

1. **If you were an obese child, you know that kids at school could be cruel.** Most of us know the feeling of being picked on in some form or fashion. I sure do. From the bus driver in first grade calling me 'big mama,' to the wretched kids in high school who missed out on getting to know a really nice person because they couldn't see past my weight, I have heard and seen it all. My kids know that in this family, we do not ever pick on, or make derogatory comments about someone's weight. My kids also know that picking on a classmate or anyone else in the world about their weight is just as big an offense as picking on them about their race, religion, sexual orientation, or anything else along those lines. Those things are just not acceptable in the Akey household.

2. **As obese teens, we missed out on things like dances and prom.** I didn't go to too many dances in school. I went to two only with a date and one with girlfriends.

Many who were morbidly obese in their young years didn't get to go to any at all. Those can be tough memories.

3. **As obese kids, we missed out on team sports and team activities.** How many of us who were obese teens got to be a cheerleader or play on the sports teams at our schools? Not too many I would guess. How many of us stayed home from trips that involved swimming and other activities that could be deemed uncomfortable or put us in a vulnerable position?

4. **As obese kids, many times we didn't get to dress like the other kids.** Kids like to fit in and feel normal. It used to really bug me that I couldn't wear a lot of the trendy styles and that certain brands of jeans just did not come in my size. As an adult, I don't think about those things, but in the mind of a teenager or pre-teen, those are important issues.

I could go on and on and on, and I am sure every single one of us has our own personal set of issues that were directly related to our being an overweight/obese child/teen. Those are memories that many of us would like to forget.

Fast forward to the present. We have chosen a path that takes us back to being healthy. For some of us, the tool of choice was surgical and for others, non-surgical. The end result is still the same. We are now a healthy and normal weight. Our diets are totally different, or at least they should be. We no longer stuff ourselves with processed garbage and empty carbs and loads of sugar. We eat fewer carbs and try to keep them complex and not simple. We eat a lot less and stay away from sweets and fast food and junk food.

This is all WONDERFUL! We feel better and look better and our labs are great. We exercise at least three times a week and are so much happier and healthier. Getting control of our health is likely the best thing we have ever done for ourselves.

I ask you this very important question now. IS THE REST OF THE FAMILY EATING HEALTHY? I realize we cannot force adults to make changes in their diets. Nothing saddens me more than hearing about situations where the spouse/partner is still eating the same garbage food they ate before the other half had weight loss surgery. I just cannot wrap my brain around a partner who sees the amazing changes in the other person and still wants to pump garbage into their own bodies. But that is another issue.

What we can control is what our kids are eating. If you lost a tremendous amount of weight, and your kids are still eating the same way, then I urge you to do some soul-searching. Dealing with unhealthy habits gets harder the older we get. Children can be taught much more easily than adults to make better choices. Why would you still feed your child fast food and snack cakes and donuts and chips and all of the same garbage food that led you to morbid obesity?

I know being a parent is hard. Ben and I have five kids between us and two are still at home. It is tough, for sure, but to me, seeing them walk in my shoes would be even tougher. Would you want your kids to suffer the same things you did as a child? Would you want them to be picked on and to miss out on activities and feel bad about themselves? Of course not! We love our children and want them to be happy.

When I was 326 pounds—my kids ate at the same places I did. We went to fast food joints and I bought a lot of snacks and snack cakes and chips and soda and junk. Once I decided to get healthy—my husband and I decided to make it a family affair. I tell people all the time that we all eat the same things. I do not cook two meals (okay, Ben does not cook two meals since he does 75% of the cooking). We all eat healthy now. Many people will look at me and roll their eyes and then proceed to tell me how that is just wrong to deprive my kids and how it just would not work with their family, etc., etc. My response to that?

BULLHOCKEY! My kids are and were no different from anyone else's. They loved fast food and loved sweets and cookies and snack cakes and soda. OF COURSE the first few weeks were hard. They fussed and asked what happened to their favorite snacks. They thought we were cruel for not buying sodas and not letting them eat at the various fast food places that are on every corner. I even had family members tell me that just because I was so fat, why did it mean I needed to deprive my kids of the goodies they love?

My first question . . . when did these goodies become accepted staples in our diets? Our parents and grandparents didn't have fast food every week and didn't have snack cakes in the house at all times. I think they turned out just fine! Oh, yes, and guess what? THEY WERE NOT AS OBESE AS OUR KIDS TODAY!

Do you even realize what you are giving your kids when you pull through that drive-through for the sake of convenience? Here are some examples for you:

McDonald's—cheeseburger, medium fries, medium Coke- 890 calories, 31 grams of fat, 1,035 mg of sodium.

Burger King—original chicken sandwich, small fries, medium Coke- 1230 calories, 60 grams of fat, 2,160 mg of sodium.

Need I say more? In the same amount of time it takes for you to drive to the fast food place, order, and take it home and eat, you could have spent that time in the kitchen with your child making a nice salad or healthy meal together and improving not just their health, but bonding with them at the same time.

It takes no more time to grab an apple from the fridge as it does to grab a Twinkie from the pantry. Which is going to help nourish your child better?

Most kids love to help in the kitchen and it is a proven statistic that kids who help their families prepare meals eat better. I am not here to make anyone feel bad, but to make you wake up and think about the things you are putting into the bodies of your kids. They deserve a healthy start and a healthy foundation. It is our job and responsibility to give that to them.

My children are NEVER rewarded with food. EVER. It has been three years since we purged the house of all of the garbage and guess what? They do not miss it at all. I asked them at dinner last night how they felt about the fact that their friends eat at fast food places quite often and their friends' parents buy sodas and cookies and all of those things and we do not. Both of them looked a little puzzled and both said they really just do not think about it anymore.

That is my point. Kids are easily trained. If you make the effort to train them to be healthier, they will do it. My kids still eat snacks after school every day. What do we keep for them? Fresh fruit, peanut butter, cheese crackers, and yes, some things I would not eat, but that are way less offensive than the sweets and garbage they used to eat. Would you rather give your child a Twinkie or a pack of peanut butter crackers?

Both of our boys at home are very athletic. Connor is s runner and even little Reed has done many 5 and 10K's with us. It didn't happen overnight and of course there were some battles in the beginning. Are our children not the most important things in our lives? Do we not want to give them the best of everything? If so, then why are we poisoning them with junk food while we try to get healthy?

My kids no longer EVER even ask to go to a fast food restaurant. Once you create a healthy habit, it tends to stick with them. They do not ask for sodas; however, occasionally when we are out to dinner, we let them order a regular Coke. It is a TREAT and not a habit. Do they eat perfectly every day? Of course not. I do not either. This is not about perfection but about making good choices one at a time that lead to better habits for a lifetime.

As a parent, why would we want to see our kids go down the road of obesity and its co-morbidities that we went down? We owe it to our kids to give them a healthy start while they are young. My good friend Dr. Connie Stapleton put it very well with this quote:

'Parents are the most influential people in their children's lives. Children are much more open to changing their habits through parental guidance. This is especially true when parents do it with them and include them in decisions. Behavior patterns are established early in life and the earlier we can establish good habits, the less difficult it will be later on. Kids inherently want to please their parents and so they are much more eager to eat healthy with their parents. Parents need to take responsibility and realize that just because kids can seem to 'get away with' eating less healthy with seemingly less adverse health effects at the time, there will come a time when the bad eating habits will catch up to them and result in similar health problems to those their parents had.'

To me, this says it all. Would you quit smoking and then allow someone to blow carcinogen-filled smoke into the face of your child? Why then, would you do all you could to fight the disease of obesity in yourself but not do all you could to prevent your children from suffering from the effects of the disease themselves?

We owe it to our kids to save them from the terrible path we took and save them from the emotional effects of being obese. I would rather see my kids upset for a few days at the new food choices than see them upset and unhealthy from a lifetime of bad food.

I promise they will thank you one day. The choice is yours. Deprive your kids of garbage food or deprive them of a lifetime of good health?" (www.bariatricguru.com)

In the weeks and months ahead, give some thought to the kinds of parents you had. Regardless of what sort of parents they were, remember, they learned to be a parent from someone as well! It's often true that we parent in many similar ways to what we learned. It's also true that people sometimes vow to do things in the exact opposite way their parents did things. Let me give you a little friendly warning—doing things in the exact opposite way of something you thought was unhealthy, is usually equally unhealthy. For example, if you weren't allowed to make any food choices for yourself as a child, but as a parent you allowed your children to eat whatever they wanted, the results would probably not be good either way!

Children need guidance, and they need boundaries. In regard to eating, our job is to teach our children what foods are healthy and to make healthy food choices before allowing for "snacks" and "desserts." It's okay to teach kids to have some of these nonessential foods, but to truly have them only from time to time and in small amounts.

We've heard about parenting and what many kids learned about eating and food in their families. What about the family backgrounds of people who grow up obese or become obese as adults? In the next chapter, we will hear more from post-ops about the families they come from.

CHAPTER FIVE

Obesity . . . An Equal Opportunity Destroyer

Food is an equal opportunity destroyer, as I like to say about all things addictive. Although this chapter is not dedicated to the addictive potential of food (trust me, that chapter's coming), there will be some references to addiction throughout this chapter as well. Obesity strikes the rich and famous (and we gloat about seeing the cellulite on the starlets, don't we ladies—somehow makes us feel better about our own human-ness). Obesity strikes the poor—and most times we feel sorry for that population who "can't afford to eat healthy foods." I realize the quotation marks make that comment seem sarcastic. It is true that many carbohydrate-rich foods like rice and pasta and potatoes go a long way toward feeding people for a little bit of money. For the percentage of the population that genuinely eats that way literally in order to feed their families rather than let them go hungry, I have tremendous compassion. For that percentage of people who uses those words as an excuse for purchasing less healthy food, but continue to take their children to eat at fast food joints several times a week, who "can't afford healthy food" but can afford smart phones and game systems and cable television, I have much less compassion. Instead, I offer this single word: *choice.*

We cannot choose what family we are born or adopted into.

We could not, as children, choose how our parents fed us. As you will see by reading contributors' information about their families, obese people are raised in a variety of environments, ranging from pretty healthy to pretty unhealthy.

Overweight and Obese Children Come from a Variety of Backgrounds:

"My parents were happily married for almost 40 years, until my father's death in 2003. Neither one had a severe weight problem like me. My mother was about 20 pounds overweight, and my father was average. I have one older brother, who was overweight as a child. Eventually he lost the weight and is average weight as an adult."

"I was the oldest of three children. My mother had multiple sclerosis, and I pretty much took care of her from the ages of 6 to 10 while my dad worked. My father put my mother in a convalescent hospital when I was 10 and we moved in with my alcoholic grandmother (his mother) and grandfather in Montana near where her hospital was. When the responsibility was taken away, I was lost. My family sort of ignored my grandmother's drinking. She was a good person, but when she drank we were pretty much on our own. My grandmother had gallbladder surgery when I was 14 and we were introduced to my dad's girlfriend in California. That Christmas, after I turned 15, my mother showed me the final divorce papers. My dad had been dating while he was married and divorced my mother while she was in the convalescent hospital. Not that she was ever going to get out of the hospital, but I felt betrayed as much as my mother must have. She cried. That January my mother came down with pneumonia and was giving up. My grandmother wouldn't let us go see her anymore (the arrangement was to see her every other Sunday). My dad married my stepmother in March of that year and they came to move us to California in July. My mother died Thanksgiving of that year. I hadn't seen my mother in 11 months. They might tell me that she died of pneumonia, but she actually died of a broken heart. She'd been abandoned.

It wasn't that I was fat but that I had an unhealthy relationship with food. It was the only thing in my life that didn't disappoint me or let me down or make me feel unloved or unwanted. I know my mother loved me. I'm not so sure about my dad, but I've always done what was expected of me—for him. My stepmother expected us to follow a very narrow line. She drank; they both drank on the weekends. I got the impression that they'd rather go to the bar than be around the house because of all of us teenagers (there were five of us now, her two daughters and us three.) She had three daughters, but her oldest had moved out. Of course there were favorites. My stepmother's two children in the home were her favorites; my sister was my dad's favorite and my brother was both their favorite."

"My parents were divorced. I was about eight when they got divorced and because my mom didn't have a job or anywhere to go, I was forced to live with my dad. I haven't mentioned it before but I also had a younger brother. He was two years younger than me. I was allowed to visit my mom every other weekend. And in sixth grade she signed me up for a dance class, which I absolutely loved. But because she was late one time, my dad kept me from visiting with her and I was forced to quit the class. I was devastated. I liked my mom and wanted to live with her.

I didn't like living with my dad and stepmom. I hated it, actually. But there wasn't anything I could do at such a young age. My mom never pursued anything because I think she was afraid of my dad, too. Back then, my dad didn't have a weight problem, but he had a drug problem. My brother wasn't overweight at all either. My stepmom was twiggy thin and struggled to keep weight on half the time. My stepdad was morbidly obese. I hated my stepmom. I shouldn't use the word hate, as it's so strong, but back when I was a kid, that's exactly what my thoughts were. My stepdad was okay. He was always nice. My brother and I got along okay when we were young. In high school, it got bumpy because he started getting into trouble."

"My parents were married for life. I was seven when my father died of a heart attack. My mother never remarried. She did the very best she could do. When my father died I was 7 and my two brothers were 12 and 17. My relationship with my two brothers was great. They protected me almost all through life. My oldest brother died last July at the age of 76. My other brother is now 72 and we are very close."

"My family is interesting. My brother and I were each adopted, so our family medical history is unknown at this time. My mom is overweight, but not obese and has continued to be active throughout her life. My dad is overweight as well and has had a hard time remaining active with bad knees. My brother has not had any weight issues."

"My parents divorced when I was 15 years old (I am now 52). It was a horrible and bitter divorce. I lived with my mother, as my father remarried a woman I hated until a few years ago when I realized she really wasn't that bad. A lot of my hatred was put into me by my jealous mother. My mom never remarried but has been with the same man for about 23 years. I have a younger brother from my parents and three half siblings from my father's second marriage. I am the oldest of all five. I didn't like my half siblings for many years due to jealousy but things are wonderful between us now. My mother has always had a weight problem and has been up and down with it forever. I have never known my father to be overweight at all. My brother (from my parents) is very overweight though."

"My mom and I have never been close. I attribute this to her getting pregnant with me when she was only 15 years old. I was always a burden to her and she would often get jealous if I got to do things that she never got to do. My social life was very limited by this. The relationship between my parents was nonexistent. They never hugged, kissed, or showed any affection towards each other. Come to think of it, they didn't show much towards us kids either.

The first time I remember my dad saying 'I love you' was the day I graduated from high school. Funny thing is, on that same day he also told me I was not really his daughter and proceeded to tell me who my real father was. I still have not talked about that with my mom and have not tried to find my real dad. I know his name and where he lives, but am afraid of being rejected by him. There is a hole in this area that someday I would like to fill, but am super-scared to take that step."

"My mother and my natural father divorced when I was about a year or so old. The man I call my father was actually my stepfather. They also divorced when I was 15 years old. There were no custody issues at the time of the divorce. My sister and I stayed with my mother. We would see our father whenever he came into town. By the time they got divorced I don't think I cared one way or the other. I was a teenager and to me it meant more freedom. By this time I was well into rebellion. I have to admit my parents did great by my sister and [me] during their divorce. We were never made to feel as if we were part of it. We were not included in the details. They were in complete agreement concerning custody and child support.

I was never made to feel as if my weight was an issue with my stepfather. My stepfather never treated me any differently than he did my sister. He really was not an involved father for the most part. Though he did start out more involved in the beginning. I remember when I was starting school he went to check out all the schools and decided which one he wanted me to go to. I remember he was there during the school functions, and we did family vacations and weekends together. I remember that the big family night out was driving over the two bridges in our town at the time (because I loved going over the bridges at night and seeing the lights) and then going out for ice cream. Another big outing was going to one of the drive-in restaurants and ordering through the car window (they did not have drive-through then). For the day-to-day stuff, he was pretty much AWOL.

I grew up with my little sister who was five years younger than me. Because of the age difference, and because of my mother, we really did not have much of a relationship, but I was always proud of her. She was the 'good' kid. The thing is, she really was the good kid!

My natural father was obese. I think this is one of the reasons my mother obsessed over my weight so much. I was a lot like him and she hated him."

As you just read, some obese people come from homes where their parents were happily married for decades. Some had parents who were divorced and remarried and created a happy home. Others came from families whose parents got remarried a number of times. Still others were raised in one-parent homes for their entire childhoods. Sometimes a parent or family member has a chronic

illness. Some obese people were only children, and others had
multiple siblings. Some obese kids felt very loved and safe in their
families; others did not. Obese people may have shared family
members who struggled with their weight or they may have fought
the battle alone. How wonderful, that in the community of WLS
post-ops, regardless of the family you grew up in, you now have an
extended family of people who definitely understand where you've
been on your road toward living at a healthy weight!

Once again, I feel compelled to make a comment (or two, or
several) that will hopefully help you understand yourself better,
whether it's now or at some time in the future. I actually need to
thank my husband for this "insert." He's been reading each chapter as I complete it; he then provides me with comments about
things he thinks I could add or delete, etc. At this particular point,
he made a suggestion about adding some material that I had
already been contemplating, but had decided to leave out of this
particular book. When he made note of the same thing, I decided
I needed to add it. So here goes:

They say that the process of going through therapy is like peeling an onion. You deal with some issue (a layer of the onion); then
it's peeled off, and lo and behold, there's another layer, which represents a different issue needing to be dealt with. You can't see
the innermost layers of the onion until you peel off the layers that
are on top of it. When people lose weight, they sometimes discover they have issues they didn't even realize because the weight
was the outer layer of the onion. As the weight comes off, they
find another layer and yet another layer of onion. You know how
people are sometimes disappointed when they lose weight and discover it didn't magically make everything in their lives happy? It's
because it wasn't just the weight (the outer layer of the onion)
causing them unhappiness. When the weight layer of the onion is
removed and they find out they're still not happy, the courageous
ones will ask, "Well, what's this next layer all about? Let's deal with

it so I can get closer to my inner happiness (which is clearly at the center of that onion)."

Let me give you an example, combining different pieces of people's stories, to illustrate what I'm talking about. I'll call the person in this example Trina. Trina is a 50-year-old woman who has a career she enjoys as a CPA. She has been married for 30 years, has two kids who are both obese, and a husband who she "adores" (noting he does work quite a few hours, but then, so does she). She comes from a "wonderful family" with parents who "loved me unconditionally." Their relationship was "pretty good,"—Dad drank "a little too much," but they remained married until death did they part.

Trina has struggled with her weight since the third grade, when she gained 30 pounds in one summer. That summer her uncle "touched her," but "that was in the past" and she insists she's dealt with it (although can't say how she's dealt with it). Trina tells the psychologist during the pre-surgical evaluation that she knows everything would be wonderful in her world if she could just get her weight off, which she has done at least two times in the past, only to gain it, and the "plus some" right along with it. The therapist suggests that it might be good for Trina to attend some counseling sessions to talk about some of the things she noted in the evaluation (dad's drinking, her uncle touching her, she and her husband working a lot, two obese kids, having lost and gained significant amounts of weight in the past)—and to help prevent her returning to food as a coping mechanism. Trina is insulted by the suggestion that she might need counseling. She was raised in a good home with plenty of love and money, she and her husband have a wonderful life with their two kids, and they both have great jobs. All she needs to do is lose this weight, and things will be great in her life. (Darned therapist . . . just wanting to get people into therapy!)

Without writing a mini-novel, let me give you a condensed version of how Trina's onion could peel away in therapy:

Onion Layer One (the problem):

"I need to lose weight . . . then I will be happy."

- Trina believes this and is not "lying" to herself or the therapist.

- Trina loses 130 pounds after WLS; she attends support group and exercises for the first six months . . . all is well in the world.

Onion Layer Two (the problem—18 months post-op):

Trina has regained 40 pounds and is no longer on top of the world.

- Trina's surgeon refers her to the psychologist (who does *not* say, "I told you so" because the psychologist knows about the onion and the fact that one layer needs to come off at a time).

- They discuss the pattern of weight regain after Trina has lost weight in the past and again now, after having WLS. Trina says her husband becomes much more interested in an "intimate relationship" when she loses weight. (She doesn't make the connection between this and the weight regain, but the therapist does.)

Onion Layer Three (the problem):

Trina was sexually abused and (subconsciously) used weight as a barrier to keep men uninterested in her sexually.

- Trina and her husband had no sexual relationship when she was at her heavy weight, but when she lost weight, he was interested in resuming that relationship.

- She was not interested in sex, which reminded her of when her uncle had molested her during the summer she was in third grade, which was also when she gained 30 pounds.

- In therapy, they talk about the sexual abuse, which, it turned out, took place because Trina's dad, who drank "a little too much," was actually a falling-down drunk on the weekends, but kept a good job during the week.

Onion Layer Four (the problem):

Dad's alcoholism resulted in his going to an inpatient treatment facility for three months following a DUI.

- Mom was therefore forced to return to work and take a second job.
- Trina and her brother went to stay with her aunt and uncle. It was the summer following third grade.
- Trina spends weeks in therapy talking about Dad's alcoholism and the toll it took on everyone in the family.

Onion Layer Five (the problem):

Trina had not felt unconditionally loved by her parents . . .

- Dad spent his time during the week working, and on the weekends he spent it in bars.
- Mom spent the weekends chasing Dad around, trying to drag him out of the bars.
- Trina felt unimportant to her parents. She spent most of her time alone on the weekends and used food as a friend.
- She was a good student and got much-needed acknowledgment from teachers for doing well in school.
- Trina spent time in therapy taking off another layer of the onion by coming to terms with the fact that there had been nothing wrong with her as a child; her parents spent their energy focused on her father's alcoholism and neglecting her needs.

Onion Layer Six (the problem):

Trina recognizes that both she and her husband spend their time focused on their careers and not one another or on their children.
- Trina becomes aware of how she had repeated the family pattern of avoiding interpersonal relationships by using a substance.
  - Her father used alcohol; she uses food.
- Trina's kids, it turned out, feel unimportant, just as Trina had.

- In therapy:
  - ○ Trina and her family work through the sadness and pain about the time they had lost with one another.
  - ○ Trina and her husband learn to have open communication and to share their thoughts.
  - ○ The entire family starts eating healthy meals together, working together to plan menus. They also begin to participate in local walks as a family.

The moral of the story here is this: Most people, like Trina, are not attempting to deny or minimize "issues" in their past or present lives. They simply aren't aware of them and/or their connection to their weight. My husband pointed this out as he was reading the stories people had sent in. He and I both attended therapy for years during our early years together and had to peel our own onions. He was noting the "minimization" of issues by some of the contributors. He wasn't judging—he's just been down the road and knows that's what we do when we're not clearly seeing the bigger picture yet.

I hope the above example helps you to see how weight often represents underlying issues; weight regain following surgery almost always indicates that underlying issues are getting in the way of being able to sustain the healthy eating and exercise activities (there are times when a physiological problem or choice of surgery affects weight loss and/or regain). We're not psychologically able to deal with all of the issues at one time; they're too overwhelming. That's why therapy can take a while. We have to peel away one layer of the onion at a time. We're not even aware that there are others underneath. I wasn't either, when I went through my own treatment program in 1989. I was just planning to get that six weeks over with and be on my happy way. *Ha!*

Just as the families of obese people are varied, the "issues" within these families are varied (and not unlike the issues in families where obesity is absent). The point of that statement is that all families have "issues." Again, the severity and number of problems within families is along a continuum, ranging from "*LOTS* of problems of many kinds" to "a few problems here and there"—(that's not a real scale—I just made it up)!

Your Peers Share the Stories of Their Families' Issues:

"My grandmother was an alcoholic. My dad, I suspect is/was an alcoholic. There were many smokers in my family, and I was a smoker, too. My grandparents were married until they died. My dad divorced my mother. My stepmother has been married three times. Her first husband abused her. I married once and divorced. I have now been married over 20 years. My sister and brother have only been married once. My oldest stepsister has been married three times. My other stepsisters have only been married once. My mother had multiple sclerosis.

When we were little (before I was 10), my parents sent us to the Church of the Nazarene on the bus. I suspected it was so that my father could sleep in on his day off and not be bothered by our 'noise.' My grandparents didn't go to church, so when we moved in with them we didn't go. My stepmother was Catholic, but we didn't go to church except on Christmas Eve, when we would go to Midnight Mass as a family. Going to church wasn't something we did as a family ever."

"My dad had a drug problem. He sold marijuana, and I know that he's done cocaine. I was actually in the room half the time and probably suffered a few contact buzzes. My mom's addiction was to food. On my dad's side, my grandma's first couple of husbands passed away. My dad's dad was actually killed in an accident when my dad was really young—like four or five. So I'm sure that some of my dad's issues could have stemmed from his own childhood.

On my mom's side, my grandparents were divorced and both remarried. Then my grandma divorced yet again after that. My grandma suffered with depression, but she never had a weight problem. She was tall and always looked fit.

I was not brought up with any sort of religion. My mom was raised Catholic, and I believe my dad's family went to Baptist church. I don't think religion was ever a part of their lives together. My dad and stepmom fought quite a bit. I had a second-floor bedroom, and I remember laying on the floor listening to them fight. They were abusive, too. I'd hear my stepmom scream and everything. I didn't like it. I was scared and therefore stayed in my room. Luckily, I never saw them . . .hearing them was bad enough for me."

"There are and were no addictions within my immediate or extended family. The only numerous divorces are mine. Two. My father passed away when I was seven. I think I was too young to be affected. I was a good kid. Never in trouble. Yes, I did attend the funeral of my father. My mother never remarried."

"My dad was an over-the-road truck driver and only came home on weekends. Every weekend was a drunk-fest, which always ended in both verbal and physical fights between my parents. Many times these fights were about affairs that my dad was having. My parents finally got a divorce when I was 18 years old."

"I come from a very long line of alcoholics. My father, his father, and his brothers were all alcoholics. My father and some of his brothers also did drugs. My mother, her father, grandfather, and one of her brothers were all alcoholics. My mother developed hepatitis and had to quit drinking, but her addictions played out in other ways. She became addicted to shopping, (grocery shopping because she could buy groceries and not feel guilty), and she also became addicted to food. She would binge on certain foods for weeks or months on end, like ice cream or Wendy's chili or McDonald's double cheeseburgers, or ham sandwiches, etc.

I really had not thought about divorces, but I guess there are many in my family. My great-grandmother divorced my great-grandfather four times. My grandmother divorced my grandfather after 40 years, my uncle was divorced, but remarried, and they have been together for almost 20 years now. My mother divorced twice and never remarried after that. I have been divorced 25 years and still haven't remarried. My sister is divorced. But there are others in the family who have been married forever. On my natural father's side, he was married three times, his parents divorced, a couple of his brothers and his sister have been divorced, some multiple times.

My uncle, who is only eight years older than I am, was in an accident when he was 17 and was in a coma with brain damage. Part of the ramifications of his accident [is] paranoid schizophrenia. I think that has had the greatest impact because he and I were more friends than niece and uncle. [Neither] of my parents passed away when I was young, but I never knew my natural father. I met him when I was 16 and then did not see him again until I was in my forties. I remember daydreaming as a child that he would come and rescue me. Needless to say, he never did.

My parents never went to church, but would send us to church on the church bus. I think they did that so they could sleep in on Sunday morning.

My parents would fight most weekends. They both drank and my father was an instigator, starting fights with other couples then not understanding why my mother would get angry. I know he hit her on several occasions, but never in front of us kids."

Although it is true a certain level of "dysfunction" exists in nearly all families, research has indicated that morbidly obese people more frequently come from homes with a history of parental loss, parental addiction of some sort, families with violence and chaos, homes where parents argued a lot, and homes in which there is often some sort of abuse. The following contributor experienced abuse at school and at home, as did many obese children:

"From the time I was three years old until my first year in college, I was a dancer, gymnast, pompom girl, and cheerleader. I wasn't obese, per se, but I was getting heavier as the years went by. In eleventh grade, my gymnastics coach taped my ankles and wrists since I was doing handsprings and flips, and putting a lot of pressure on my joints. I stopped gymnastics after eleventh grade but continued to dance. I am a trained ballet, tap, and jazz dancer. It was the kind of dance you saw on the original show Fame.

I tried track and field but I was not a runner, so I did shot-put. That was a joke because I wasn't very good at all. I even made the swim team but then I had to swim laps, and, well . . . I was just not a long distance anything. LOL. Track, swim, etc. So . . . I went to the diving team. That was as good as shot-put, so I became the swim team pseudo manager. I wanted to be a part of something so much. I really was, though. I was a dancer. I was a good dancer. I could've been a great dancer had I continued. As I got older, I could still dance like I used to, but I felt it wasn't as attractive to watch anymore. . . . (Now that I've lost weight, I'm dancing again, and I love it as much as I did when I was doing my very last dance, *A Chorus Line.*)

I had no physical limitations growing up. My folks always encouraged me to try out or be something. My mother was wonderful like that. She was a dancer and a theater actress as well, so it was wonderful for her to come watch me. And, even show me some moves. My (new) dad put a violin in my arms in sixth grade, as he was a wonderful violinist. I, sadly, failed miserably at violin, but I do play drums, piano, and now guitar. Not well, just for fun. I'm what's called a party favor. I can play *Kumbaya* at a campfire or 'Lean on Me' on the piano in a huge group, but shh . . . don't listen too closely, or you'll see that I'm playing by ear! LOL. My entire family was musical—dancing, acting, singing. It was my dad who gave me an appreciation for classical music and for my favorite, a Latin opera called Carmina Burana. I remember lying on the floor by these really HUGE speakers and singing along. Now, remember, this was in Latin. But I still sang my heart out while it played. My dad taught me to love classical music and my mom taught me to love Paul Anka and fifties music. My sister tried to get me to love the Grateful Dead, but I was grateful I was into Barry Manilow, Leif Garret, and Shawn Cassidy. LOL!

I wasn't very social when I was young. My parents ALWAYS knew, if I fought not to go to a dance, for instance, to make me go anyway. They knew once I was there, I'd have the best time. I honestly cannot remember a time they were incorrect about that. Even today, I'll call my Ma 3,000 miles away and tell her I don't want to go somewhere, and she'll say, 'Go. You know once you're there, you'll have a great time.' And she's always right. My mother is always right.

I have a funny memory of being about eight or nine in Harrisburg, Pennsylvania. I must quietly admit that I looked IDEN-TICAL to Danny Partridge. LOL. One day I was with a friend walking to the Jewish Community Center, and we asked a man what time it was. (Honest to goodness, this can't be more true, and I chuckle as I write it.) His reply was exactly this: 'It's 2:00 p.m., son.' He smiled and left. My friend and I were on the grass in hysterics. He really thought I was a boy. But, I seemed to love it.

My real friends never teased me when I was a kid. In high school, though, the jocks would say cruel things to me. Some of them would call me fat, but mostly, they just had nothing to do with me. Now, don't get me wrong. I was in gymnastics with a few of the jocks; they were the coolest and we were extremely close back then. But they weren't the 'football jocks.' Those guys that lined the halls every single morning and afternoon were the ones that weren't the nicest to me. Looking back, though, I wasn't fat. I just wasn't a size 0. But I wore my shirts tucked in, jeans, etc. They didn't have to know I got them at the ONLY plus size store in all of Maryland. (This was in the seventies.) I never dressed out of style.

This is a story I have shared with a few people but not many. My Ma remarried when I was going into sixth grade. I loved that school, and I made a ton of friends. Then all hell broke loose and I was sent to a private Jewish School. I was away from my new friends and was put with people that had been together since kindergarten. I was a tomboy. Hardcore tomboy and all the boys in seventh grade would play with me. I'd be picked for baseball team, basketball, etc. I was playing 'king of the hill' one day with all the boys. (We didn't have electronics back then . . . well, we had Pong. . . .) The principal came out and very loudly put a stop to it. He called me out and into his office. He then said he was calling my parents to come in. He told me that I could not play with the boys anymore. I had breasts, and the boys would hurt me. He said a lot more, but I didn't listen. My heart broke from that moment, because I knew in the girls' locker room, they were going to let me have it. They were jealous because I was as good at sports as the boys and they were just—well—girls that looked pretty. And, they did let me have it, too. In the locker room, the girls made fun of me, as I expected. I had developed in seventh grade in all the right places, and these girls were mostly flatter than an ironing board, yet they felt compelled to humiliate me and embarrass me for having hair where they didn't and having little breasts where they only had dots.

I never really knew how to fight back, but I do remember this one thing. It was the first time in my life that I wanted to die. I had always been 'one of the boys' for as far back as I could remember and this principal put a stop to it and made me feel ashamed.

My mother, and at that time, stepfather, always did a great job making sure we had the correct meals. Back then it was meat of some kind, vegetables, and one fun item (mashed potatoes, etc.), and then dessert. We always got to have dessert, unless I was bad. LOL. Which was a lot."

"Since I wasn't an obese child, there were really never any weight comments. Ever. However, when I got older (after age eight, I think) the comments began. They were from my grandfather (who I loved more than anyone else in the entire world), my grandmother, and once in a while my uncle teased me. But, he, like my grandpa, was my hero. So, anything he or Grandpa said, I tried to do and please them. I never succeeded. Even to this day.

I remember being told that obesity was in my genes and I'd better be careful. I never listened. I didn't care. My Nana, (my biological dad's mother) used to tell me over and over, 'You have such a beautiful face. If you would just lose weight, you could find a man and be happy.' I just figured I'd be alone forever, because no one would want me fat. How did I deal with THAT? I ate more.

Food was a big issue in my home from age 10 on. Food was used as a punishment and also as a threat. The sorts of things I heard about food are as follows (keep in mind, I'm talking about circa sixties and seventies): 'Eat everything on your plate; there are children starving in Africa,' or 'If you don't stop playing with your food, I'm taking it away and you can go to bed. Without dinner.' It was no secret that I would NEVER put a lima bean in my mouth, yet they were still put on my plate to eat. I ended up using the Africa comment as a stand-up joke: 'I was told all about the kids in Africa starving and I had to eat. I'm still not sure what THAT had to do with them being hungry but I said, 'Look Ma, I ate for those kids AND their entire country. They're still hungry and I'm fat. Really?' Needless to say, that joke went over very well! ☺ (I did stand-up for seven years as a plus-size lady.)

I do not recall ever having a CHOICE whether or not to finish my food. I had to. And, I still think that today. I still think I must finish all of my food. Every celebration included food. Passover

Seder was the best because I could SNEAK whatever I wanted (including alcohol), and no one paid attention. There were so many of us. I do believe I became a food addict long before I knew what it was. As I grew, food was my comfort, along with other things, but food always. If I ate, I felt nothing but full. Or not. If I was sad, I felt nothing but full. Or not. You get the picture. Being Jewish, food is a part of all rituals. Funerals—OMG— the food is amazing. (Sorry.) Weddings—wow—a foodie's haven!

The ONLY people in my family who were not overweight were my little sister, one uncle, and my grandpa. All the rest of us (mostly the women, sans my little sister until recently) were overweight or obese. The men, not so much. My uncle, now that he's in his 60s, has battled his weight. My sister had three sons, starting 13 years ago, and it saddens me that she's gaining weight. The one thing I don't want in life is for her to have to be like I was. She's so beautiful and has such a wonderful spirit AND family. But we don't talk weight. My mother is very heavy and getting heavier, is diabetic, and getting other weight-related illnesses. It's very scary to me because she's very stationary.

I have a recollection of seeing my biological father when he came to town. I was so excited. I hadn't seen him in a long time and wanted to look perfect. I went shopping the night before and got the prettiest outfit. I knew he was going to take me to a nice restaurant. I made sure my hair was perfect, too. When I walked into the room, my father was on the phone with his son. The only thing I remember him saying was, 'I have to go. Godzilla just walked in.' I have no more words to add to this.

A big thing for me throughout my childhood was not feeling safe or protected. I felt physically threatened and defenseless. This lack of protection led to feelings of insecurity and unworthiness. Food was a great source of comfort.

In spite of it all, I grew up happy. I was a difficult kid. I had ADHD, but they didn't know how to diagnose that yet. My only sibling, my younger sister, was a charm. I, however, was a handful. I give my mother a lot of credit. I don't tell her that enough, but I do. I was a lot to handle and if using food as a punishment worked, so be it. However, it led to me sneaking food.

As far back as I can remember, once my sister and I moved to Pennsylvania, we'd have our dinner and when it was bedtime, I'd always make her go out and sneak us food. Always. It was just never enough for me. I could never seem to eat enough. My mother ALWAYS told me that I could do whatever I put my mind to doing. My dad was the one that said I needed an education. I tried that for one year (in college) and failed miserably. I was just never a student and I always wanted to 'just be a writer, so no college was needed.' To this day, my folks are my biggest supporters. My mom will be the one that will have to be restrained when I get my Emmy or Oscar. LOL.

As I said, I always had a lot of friends. But, starting from age seven, everyone I began to love and care for, would leave. Either by moving (not my choice as a child) or they'd move. As I grew older, that pattern was apparent in all aspects of my life. The worst was that I never got to say goodbye. I never, ever had closure.

That brings me to adulthood and the same behavior. Example: I was removed from school in the middle of second grade in West Virginia and taken to Pennsylvania and put into the private Jewish School. I did have a few friends since I was always visiting my grandparents in Harrisburg, but it did take a little time to adjust. The point is, I never said goodbye to my friends in West Virginia. Then, after four years, I was to go to summer camp and when it was over, I was uprooted to Rockville, Maryland, when my mom remarried. Again, I never had closure or said goodbye to all the kids I'd been in school with until the end of fifth grade. Then, I went to sixth grade, made friends, and was moved to a school where I knew no one again. Back to school in eighth grade where I was finally with the people I would spend the rest of my school years. That pattern of not having closure, as I mentioned, has followed me to this day. No closure. As I got older, I would say, 'They left me,' but I had to look at my behavior. I left THEM. I would leave before they could leave me because I thought it would hurt less. That was never the case.

I never felt left out of activities when I was young, but as a young adult, I did. My friends would go skiing, riding horses, go to amusement parks, etc. You get the idea. I always made excuses not to go. Or I'd go and then watch them, saying I couldn't do this or that. Or I'd say I was afraid. My real friends knew. My real friends wouldn't ask me to do those things. In the past, I always surrounded myself with people I loved unconditionally and who loved me back the same way. I was lucky to have the friends I had when I was growing up. I still have a couple of them, and I cherish them like precious gold.

Here's the thing. I didn't become AWARE that being fat was

something to be ashamed of or angry about. I just didn't pay attention, really. I don't think so. I'm speaking about me as a child. Not after college. My mom and dad split when I was seven. She remarried when I was going on 10. My stepdad adopted my sister and even though I was almost 18, it was what I wanted.

My biological father lives on the east coast. I think I'm pretty much a huge disappointment to him, and it's hard for me to talk about it. I rarely saw him when I was young. He flew me to California when I was 16 and sent me packing early because I had apparently lied to people he knew. When I was older and moved to L.A., he was local, but we just never really saw each other. Now he's back east, and we don't really have much of a relationship. I love him very much, and I'm a lot like him. I'm proud of that, but it's too late for us to reconcile. I know he wanted more from me regarding a career, etc. Both my sister and stepbrother are educated and are now educators. I'm neither.

I always ate. Happy, sad, miserable, mean, loving—didn't matter. I grew up Jewish. Eat everything on your plate. EVERYTHING. Or I had to sit there till I finished. To me, that's abuse. I had RNY and I'm still eating badly at times, but losing. I'm a work in progress."

The next chapter is the one dedicated to addiction, but perhaps you have already noticed that many of the contributors have had alcohol or drug addiction issues in their immediate and/or extended families. Many of them had families where obesity was prevalent in the family as well. Food, like alcohol and drugs, can be an addiction. One that is carried out in a lot of families, but is often ignored as an addiction.

Difficulties in the home, whether they are caused by nature (parental illness or death, disruption due to hurricanes or other natural disasters) or whether the problems are the result of alcohol, drugs, or simply having unhappy parents, children suffer the effects. Overeating is sometimes a way children escape the difficulties of living in an unpleasant atmosphere. The resulting obesity can cause another set of problems all its own. Here are some additional comments contributors made about being an obese child:

"As a child I never felt good enough, and yet I felt as if every-one counted on me to stay strong and do what was expected of me. Food was the only thing that never left and never judged and never let me down. Now I know I'm addicted to sugar and I know at any minute I could let it conquer me again. I'm motivated never to let that happen again."

"Throughout my childhood, I feared my dad and suffered his teasing. Because my mom never really did anything, I eventu-ally came to believe that I was fat and would be fat. I didn't find comfort in food until high school. And then the emotional eat-ing continued beyond that. I can say though that since surgery . . . I feel as though I'm completely healed of that. I've found self-confidence and self-worth and I'm healing. I'm living again. I love and appreciate life. Thanks for allowing us a chance to share our stories."

"I had a good childhood. My mother loved all her boys and took very good care of us. I just like food. . . . What can I say. . . ."

"I tried so many times to lose weight. Weight Watchers, Atkins, boot camp. You name it, I tried it. I believed RNY gastric bypass was my only solution. I was approved for the surgery and had it on July 14, 2010. I had some complications with my sur-gery. I ended up having a bowel obstruction and then an internal infection. I was in the hospital for 19 days. Why did I do this to myself? I have lost over 100 pounds and continue to lose. I weigh less than I did when I graduated high school. I am getting my eating habits under control. I do not go out to eat, unless it is a special occasion now. I spend less money on food, but now spend on new clothes. I am so happy to be alive and thank God every day for giving me this new outlook on life and a fresh start to actually live my life."

"I really feel that food was my best friend throughout my child-hood; it really helped me through all the negativity in my family, especially with my parents arguing all the time and through their divorce. I always knew that the food would be there for me no matter what the time or the weather was. I could always rely on that source of comfort."

"I was a miserable child and teenager. As a teenager I would go between starving myself to accommodating and rebelling. It is just within the last year that I have learned to love and accept myself for who I am and I will be 51 in March. It has been a long road but I am happy to have made it. I am now trying to repair all the damage that dieting and overeating did to my metabolism and health. I have made peace with my childhood and my mother, and I have forgiven those who abused me. More importantly, I have forgiven myself. I have come to love the woman I am. I understand all that I have been through is the reason I am who I am today."

In *Breaking Free from Emotional Eating*, Geneen Roth talks about eating in response to whatever pain we endured as children: "There isn't enough food in the world to heal the isolation of those years. There isn't enough food to fill the space created by the deprivation and the ensuing feelings of craziness."

As noted at the beginning of this chapter, we had no choice about what family we were born or adopted into. We could not, as children, choose how our parents fed us. And although we develop habits related to eating and other behaviors from the families we grew up in, as adults we have the ability to *choose to change* any negative attitudes and behaviors we learned and implement positive practices instead. We also have the *choice* to peel the onion that made up our life and uncover any abuse or other issues from our past in order to move forward with the emotional freedom to keep the weight off and fully enjoy life.

CHAPTER SIX

Food and Abuse—What's the Connection?

Sadly, many, many obese people were the victims of some sort of abuse at various times in their lives. You read many passages in the two previous chapters about the many different forms. The following contributor portrays how weight can serve as an emotional protector. As this woman wisely notes, using food and weight to provide emotional protection is usually a subconscious process that serves an important purpose. In the process of losing weight, she has been able to recognize the "purpose" her weight played in her life, which was to protect her. The safer she begins to feel in her adult life and the more she learns to loves herself, the less need she has for weight to keep her "safe."

"My fat cocoon: My subconscious obesity cocoon began when I was a young girl around the age of 11. I was the daughter of an alcoholic father and a very hardworking—sometimes three jobs at a time—mother who was trying to keep her family afloat and together.

My mom was working all the time, and my dad worked off and on. So, it fell to him to watch my two younger brothers and me. But, most of the time, the responsibility of watching my brothers was delegated to me. My youngest brother, then just a baby, was all my responsibility. I had to grow up fast. I developed quite early, physically, as well. I began to show the shape and figure of a well-developed teenager at the age of 11. I was quite the cutie at that age.

Boys started showing me attention, of course. More attention than I knew what to do with and more than I could handle. For the most part, they were all older boys. In one case there was a much older teenager—maybe 16 or 17 at that time—and he wanted to be my 'boyfriend.' He made advances toward me and told me that's what it meant to be 'going together.' At my age, with no education from my parents on this matter, I knew no better. So I thought this was the way it was supposed to be. He continued making his advances. Another time a young man, who lived next door, made his advances. This continued with a lot of boys on our street. And all of these boys/men always wanted to be my 'secret' boyfriends. Duh! Here's your sign. But, again, I did not know any better. Where were my parents to teach me self-worth?

One day the brother of one of my so-called boyfriends, along with three of his friends, decided to wait for me at the end of the road we lived on. At the end of the road was an old outhouse. I walked this road with friends on a daily basis. But on this day my friends couldn't go when I could, so I went alone. As I neared the church, these boys were waiting for me. I knew them all, so I thought nothing of it.

They hollered at me to come and see what they had found. So, I went over to see what it was. As I neared the area around the outhouse, the boy I thought was the 'cutest' was in the outhouse. He said, 'It's in here.' As I got closer to the door, the other three pushed me in and locked the door from the outside. So, here I was, locked in there with him. I asked him where it was. And he then started to try and reach under my shirt. I pulled away as far as I could, but he was stronger, and I could not go anywhere. Then he started for my shorts. I began to struggle more and started to cry, all along asking him, between sobs, 'Why are you doing this?'

The Lord was really watching over me, because just when he had gotten my shorts down and was beginning to get my panties down, my friend came looking for me. And like kids do, she was yelling at the top of her lungs. Well, this scared the three boys outside, so they unlocked the door, which I didn't know at the time that they had. And they headed down the road. As they passed my friend she asked them if they had seen me. They said they had seen me with their friend around the church. So, she proceeded the rest of the way, yelling at the top of her lungs, which scared the boy who was inside the outhouse with me.

He pulled his pants up and headed down the road. She asked him where I was, and he said I was by the church. By the time she reached me, I had pulled my clothes back on and had gotten out of that place and was beginning to walk home.

She could tell that I had been crying and asked me what was wrong. Of course, being ashamed, I did not want to tell her anything. She persisted as we walked home together. So I told her the whole thing.

She was furious and went and told her older sister. She, in turn, came to me and explained that they were in the wrong and I should tell my parents. 'Tell my parents!' I exclaimed! No, not in a million years. She persisted and told me that if I did not tell them by the next morning, she was going to. And I knew she meant every word of what she had said. So, I waited until the last minute and told my parents. At first they did not believe me. Then my friend backed me up. They were furious and wanted names.

All during this I felt as if I were to blame. It felt like I was carrying the guilt of the world on my shoulders. My parents called the police, so again I had to tell this horrifying story, and again, I felt the same guilt and shame. They contacted the four boys and their parents. Of course they denied it at first. Then they came up with the untrue story that I had asked them to meet me up there, and I was the one teasing and wanting to have sex with them.

'How could they lie?' were my thoughts, but they remained only thoughts. For that was the place of women and girls. The police told them and their parents that they were to have NO contact with me whatsoever or they would be charged with attempted rape. And to this day there have been no charges. There was no contact, other than the occasional 'Hi' to each other after we graduated high school. They all ended up in trouble for one thing or another eventually. But, in the meantime, via their mouths, I was labeled easy, a slut, a whore, etc.

Around the same time that this was going on, my dad started paying a lot of unwanted attention to me. The leers, the stares, the comments on my developing body, attempts to get me to do things that a father and daughter should not do. I managed to avoid having sex with him. But there was a constant fear in me when he was around. I avoided him at all costs. This was not the way a daughter should feel about her father. I avoided him until I was 18, married, and moved out. But there was still that fear, an ever-present fear. And it lasted for many more years. I think until his death. I managed to grow inside and forgive him, but still had a little voice inside that told me to be cautious. I guess I forgave him but I kept my guard up. I still wanted to hide in my little cocoon, wrapped up in my safe, little home. My sanctuary.

My emotions were so crazy at that time. I was trying to avoid my dad, I was hurt, scared, confused, and filled with hate. I hated him, but most of all I hated myself. And I didn't know why I hated myself. Later on, I figured out that I hated what these males had done to me—not the sinner but the sin, so to speak.

Not too long after that, my neighbor, my 'friend,' attempted to have sex with me. What was wrong with me? Why did men want to hurt me? What was I doing wrong? I shut down. I hated myself, my body, and everyone else that crossed my path. I was scared to be left alone with my dad. I avoided him and every other male that that had attempted to have sex with me. I was labeled once again, slut, whore, easy, and every other slang word they could think of. I was accused by my parents of being on drugs. And they accused others of slipping drugs in my drinks or food. I didn't think my mom would believe me about any of the things my dad had attempted. As I grew older, I vowed to never tell her about my dad's advances. And I never did. She died not knowing how cruel he was and how scared I was of him. As far as I know, she never figured it out.

I felt she had enough to deal with: his abuse of her sexually, physically, and emotionally. He not only abused me and my mom, but my brother, a middle child. My brother turned to alcohol, drugs, and sleeping around because of it, and he is still out in the world. I have very little contact with him. He is NOT dealing with any of his abuse from his childhood. I'll continue to pray for him but cannot allow myself to relive my childhood through him. I cannot let him abuse my love for him as a brother by using me or relying on me for his addictions. I will not be his enabler like my mom was for my dad.

Now, around the same time, two major events happened to me, the first being that someone invited me to church. I got saved and knew what it meant. I had to walk to the church to be able to go, and I eventually quit. But, the Lord was still with me and watching over me, even though I was not allowed to go to church anymore. It was too much of an inconvenience to my parents. I ended up turning my back on God. But, I now know that these things that had happened to me were wrong. The second important event was that I started to put layers on my cocoon, my safe haven. Just like the caterpillar spins layers on his cocoon. But, my layers were made of fat.

I can remember my first binge-eating episode like it was yesterday. It was at my grandparents' house. This is where we went on Sunday instead of my parents letting me go to church, where I thought the Lord was. I didn't know that I carried Him in my heart with me everywhere I went. I felt safe at my grandparents' house. My dad would not dare attempt anything there, and he never did. One Sunday, after yet another remark or stare during the week is when I started to layer my cocoon with food. I ate so much cornbread, brown beans, and coleslaw, not to mention anything else I could manage to eat, that I was sick within an hour. (My grandma was a wonderful cook.) I cried and whined until my parents couldn't stand it anymore. My dad gave me paregoric, and I had no sooner gotten out of bed when I started throwing up. That was the first big layer of food that I laid on my body. It felt good to eat. I had control. No one could stop me from doing it. Even if I had to sneak and do it. And I became a 'pro' at that.

I never became a bingeing bulimic, but I purged in other ways. For example, exercise. As far as being anorexic, I would not eat for short periods of time but never for too long because Lord knows I love to eat. It makes me feel safe, warm, and in control. Eventually, I just gave up all of the exercise and periods of not eating. I just started eating uncontrollably.

Layer after layer of fat added on to my cocoon. Subconsciously I knew that if I were fat enough, no one would pay attention to me in that way, the 'bad' way. But by the time I started adding these layers, I was already married to my wonderful husband (who, by the way, saved me from the life my brother is leading now). But there was nothing he could do about my food addiction. It helped that he was overweight, partly my doing, as he ate with me. It made me feel better about myself and my food addiction. Now, I am not saying he is a food addict. He just allowed me to fuel my addiction. He didn't understand it any more than I did at that time.

Connie Stapleton, PhD

All my adult life I played the yo-yo dieting game. Up and down, up and down. And still didn't know why. All I knew was that I hated my body—thin or fat. It was ugly, disgusting, and I hated it. I can remember times when my husband and I made love that I would turn over and cry, wondering the whole time how could he make love to me, as I was FAT. Notice I didn't say have sex, I said make love. I knew there was a difference. And I knew that we didn't have S-E-X. We made love. Poor man—he has put up with so much in my journey. He has been an absolute angel in my life. And I love him more and more each day. We have been together for 30 years this year. All due to his patience and the love he has for me. He has been my rock.

I soon found Overeaters Anonymous and was indirectly 'reintroduced' to my Lord. I came to realize that He had never left me, but that I left Him. I eventually lost some weight, but soon the group dissolved and again I started putting the fat layers right back on. More up and downs. Depression hit me hard. More layers. I neglected my God, my husband, my sons, and myself. Always putting myself last on the list.

Now, to bring you to about 10 years ago. Happily married, a pastor's wife, both sons married, and grandchildren. Both sons are preachers—one being a pastor. A perfect life but still I hated my body. A lady in our church had weight problems and had RNY surgery. After our talks I knew this was going to be my way out of this cocoon I had spun for myself. But at that time I had no insurance. My doctor recommended that I file for disability. Yet another reason to hate myself and my body.

I was no longer able to carry my weight, and the weight was damaging my health. My 'layers' had made me disabled. After about two years I finally received my disability benefits. Now I had the label of being 'disabled.' With that label came medical insurance. But of course it did not cover gastric bypass surgery. Two years later I heard rumors that the insurance did occasionally cover this surgery under certain circumstances. So, after another six months or so of thinking, researching, praying, and enduring numerous emotional ups and downs, I thought I would look into the surgery option some more. I talked with several people about their surgery experiences and, of course, got mixed opinions. One lady gave me the number of one of the most caring surgeons I have ever met. I called and got the place and time of his next mandatory seminar. After the seminar, I was convinced, my husband was convinced, and my new doctor, who had had RNY surgery five years prior, was convinced that this was my only way back to a healthy body. Not necessarily thin but healthy.

So I started my pursuit of my gastric bypass surgery. Of course, my insurance company denied me, not only once, but twice. I was going crazy, and the layers kept piling on. I asked my doctor to write a letter to the insurance company, advice from a dear friend I met on the WLSFA.org. page, and by golly, it worked. She had done it. She convinced them it was a life-or-death situation. After five months of fighting, begging, crying, and pleading with the insurance office, it was all worth it. I was approved and scheduled for surgery within two weeks. I was again an emotional wreck, even though I knew this was the right thing to do. I got through that little meltdown and had my surgery the next morning. I went through my surgery with no complications and seemed to heal quite easily. I was up and going in just one week. Not fast, mind you, but I was up and going. I had my surgery on Monday and the next Sunday I was sitting in my seat at church.

Now—losing the weight has not been easy. I have struggled. I have been going through a lot of emotions. I still want to eat for comfort at times. I have to watch what I eat. I have to exercise. I have to keep a positive attitude. I have to get better. I do have dumping syndrome when I eat too much or when I eat something that just happens not to agree with me for that meal. It is never the same thing, it seems like. But I do not dump with sugar, my weakness. I wanted to dump with this particular thing. I am managing not to eat much sugar. I made the mistake of testing it and wish I had never done it. But I can't dwell on that. I just have to stay away from it and keep it out of my house.

I am in contact with people on weight loss pages daily. This is another tool that I use. My biggest tool is my RNY surgery. My biggest supporter is my husband. He wants nothing more than for me to be happy and healthy. I have met some resistance before and after my surgery. My brother and his wife didn't think I should have it done. My daughter-in-law, who I thought was one of my biggest supporters, told me she thought it was 'a chicken's way out to become bulimic and/or anorexic.'

Some people are shocked that I had the surgery; some are proud of me for having the courage to do it. I have been very surprised with all the different feedback I have gotten. I just recently decided to tell people about my surgery. I've kept it a secret from most people. But I no longer care what they think of me. They can take me the way I am or leave me alone. It is still an emotional rollercoaster at times, but worth it to get myself healthy again and to learn how to love myself for who I am. Thin, fat, fluffy, big boned, or any other label I have had put on me for my whole life. I am losing weight, not as fast as I want to, but slow is better. I am peeling off the layers of my cocoon just like I put them on. I am seeing a beautiful butterfly emerge from her fat cocoon. She will continue to peel the layers off and emerge to be the butterfly she was meant to be.

Thank you, Lord, for this gift of a new life you have given me. Amen

Cocoon begone!"

Abuse comes in many forms. Sadly, when one is a child and experiences some sort of abuse, he or she may not recognize it as such because it is the norm in the household. For example, if children are criticized on a regular basis, they aren't even aware that it is taking place, perhaps until they observe other parents speaking kindly and encouragingly to their kids. In my very large, extended family, every adult smoked, drank, and had quite a "potty mouth." So it wasn't just in my home, but in the homes of the people we socialized with throughout my childhood. I just thought that when you grew up, you smoked, drank, and had a foul mouth. And I followed right along in those footsteps! Fortunately, I've given up two of the three (if you've been around me for any length of time, you might hear the potty coming from my mouth)!

In one of my favorite books of all time, *Adult Children: The Secrets of Dysfunctional Families*, by John Friel, PhD, he outlines various forms of abuse. The following information is from his book. Look it over and please keep an open mind as you read it. Sadly, people want to excuse the people in their lives who have hurt them. Perhaps even more sadly, people want to blame the abuser's behavior on themselves, noting they "deserved it." This is not the first layer on the onion—it sometimes takes a while to accept that children do not deserve any form of abuse. But that's another book. For now, read through the information about forms of abuse. When you're finished reading this book, order Dr. Friel's!

Emotional Abuse and Neglect (Examples):
- Blaming the child
- Altering a child's reality (intellectual abuse) e.g., "Dad's not drunk and passed out; he's just tired"
- Overprotecting, smothering, excusing, blaming others for the child's problem
- Double messages: "Of course, I love you, dear" (as Mom tenses up and grits her teeth)
- Not talking about the abuse at all.
- Failure to nurture, care for, or love the child
- Failure to provide structure or set limits
- Not listening to, hearing, or believing the child
- Expecting the child to provide emotional nurturing to the parents, to make the parents feel good
- Not being emotionally present due to mental illness, chemical dependency, depression, or compulsivity
- Failure to encourage educational or intellectual development

Physical Abuse and Neglect (Examples):
- Slapping, shaking, scratching, squeezing, hitting, beating with boards, sticks, belts, kitchen utensils, yardsticks, electric cords, shovels, hoes
- Throwing, pushing, shoving, slamming against wall or objects
- Burning, scalding, freezing
- Forcing of food or water, starving

- Having to watch others be physically abused
- Overworking
- Denying food, clothes, shelter
- Leaving the child alone in age-inappropriate ways
- Leaving a child who is too young in charge of others
- Failure to provide medical care
- Allowing or encouraging the use of drugs, alcohol
- Failure to protect the child from the abuse of others, including spouse

Verbal Abuse and Neglect (Examples):
- Excessive guilting, blaming, shaming
- Name-calling, put-downs, comparisons
- Teasing, making fun of, laughing at, belittling
- Nagging, haranguing, screaming, verbal assault

Sexual Abuse and Neglect
- Sexual abuse occurs most frequently when children are between the ages of 9 and 12, but it also occurs with regularity in infancy, which makes it extremely difficult for a recovering person to ever identify and deal with it.
- Fondling, touching, innuendos, jokes, comments, looking, leering
- Exposing self to, masturbating in front of, mutual masturbation
- Oral sex, anal sex, intercourse, penetration with fingers or objects
- Stripping and sexual punishments, enemas
- Pornography—taking pictures or forcing the child to watch
- Forcing children to have sex with each other
- Not teaching children about sex—not talking about puberty, menstruation, nocturnal emissions, etc.

Vicarious Abuse

- Vicarious abuse is a special case of abuse, in which the victim is part of a family or other system in which someone else is abused in some way. This type of abuse can be just as damaging as actually being the recipient of the other types of abuse listed above.

Abuse and Neglect Result in:

- Perfectionism
  - Unrealistic expectations for self or others
  - Perfectionism grows out of unhappiness and is the breeding ground for constant criticism. Constant criticism is the surest way to leave a child with a deep sense of worthlessness and shame.
  - People who grow up in critical families internalize those messages so that when they enter adulthood, they unconsciously do the same thing to themselves. A little voice inside of them will always be saying, "This isn't good enough. You're not doing it right. There's something wrong with you."

- Rigid Rules/Belief Systems
  - There is only one right way to be. There is only one right way to do it. I must be in control at all times or my life will topple. An awful lot of compulsive behavior and obsessive thinking comes under this heading.

- **Don't Talk, and Keep Secrets**
  - "Don't air dry your dirty laundry in public" is the battle cry of dysfunctional families.
  - In dysfunctional families, this rule means "Don't yell for help when you're about to drown." It means little children must go to school every day, smiles on their faces and knots in their stomachs, because they have been up half the night listening to their parents have a bloody battle over money, or alcohol, or in-laws. It means those same children dare not to try to share their pain with a friend or a school counselor because

if they do, they will be emotionally or physically beaten or shamed for sharing "family secrets" outside the family. Above all, it means that we will grow up to believe that we must handle all of our problems by ourselves, alone, in isolation.

- Inability to Play/Have Fun
- Denial

  ○ Denial is one of the ways that we protect ourselves from a reality that is too painful for us to let into our conscious minds. It serves a healthy purpose as well as an unhealthy one, depending upon how we use it.

Thank you, Dr. John Friel, for your remarkable wisdom and for sharing it in your books.

Tragically, many obese people have been the victims of sexual abuse. Rosemary and Connie valiantly spoke up about this in the WLSFA documentary that inspired this book. Many of the other contributors courageously shared their stories of this dreadful reality:

"Hmmm, abuse . . . always a hard one to talk about. I am a victim of sexual abuse. Two uncles, two cousins, and my dad all took their turns abusing me from about age six until sometime in junior high when I finally got up the courage to stop them. I have done a little bit of counseling and am not sure if more would help. Just seems like one of those things that happens to most all girls and we just try to forget about it."

"I was sexually abused by my grandfather around the age of six or seven. I ate to comfort myself and now find that I still eat when I am emotional. I eat to avoid my emotions. I discovered later in my life that I was a food addict. I didn't talk about the abuse till my twenties. Then later in my adult life I got some counseling about it. During my childhood, I don't know if I felt safe or not. I do know I felt insecure and unworthy. I did not think I was liked by guys or fit the Barbie doll image. I was brunette, I did not have long legs, and I wasn't thin. My sister was like a Barbie doll, and my mom was too. I was always told I looked like my dad. My dad was tall and thin, but I did not want to look like my dad (no offense, Dad); I wanted to look pretty like my mom! I wasn't unattractive; I just felt that way.

During my pre-op counseling, and then after I had surgery, I always tried to figure out why I had so much trouble with my weight. It seemed hard for me to figure it out until I had lost about 80 pounds and was starting to feel better about the way I looked. I started my day with a bike ride and had two different guys make sexual comments. This really creeped me out. The next day I went for a run and wore compression pants and a fitted top. Again I had a guy make a comment and felt like everyone was looking at me. I literally broke down and got back to my car as soon as possible. I hated it! I hated them! I sat in my car and cried and cried. I wanted to be fat again! I wanted them to stop look-ing at me! At that moment I knew that being fat was my comfort zone so that men wouldn't pay attention to me. I am sure this is because of the sexual abuse.

I am only 18 months post-op now and am at my goal weight of 140 pounds. I have gone to counseling concerning this inse-curity. The counseling along with support from my wonderful husband is helping me deal with this. I am starting to feel better about the way I look and don't feel quite so self-conscious when I wear something a little 'sexy.' I feel healthier now than I can ever remember and would not change my choice to have RNY surgery for anything!"

"I was sexually abused beginning at the age of four over a period of years by a caretaker's son. There were three of us girls who were staying with this person, and he would take turns abusing us at night. Two of us tried to tell his mother what he was doing, and we were beat with an old pink Avon brush and sent to bed with nothing to eat for the rest of the day and night. She told us we were nasty little girls. I was then raped by a family friend when I was 12. It actually happened about two weeks before I started my period for the first time. I was terrified that I was going to be pregnant. From the ages of 12 to 16, I was molested by another family friend and by my uncle, too many times to count. When I turned 16 I put an end to it all. . . .

I have since come to realize that the sexual abuse, along with the emotional abuse from my mother played a huge part in my becoming obese. Yes—I ate for comfort, but more than that my obesity subconsciously became my shield. I hid behind a mountain of fat. It's funny, but the bigger you are, the more invisible you become. For me it was a way to keep people at arm's distance. I didn't have to let anyone in because no one wanted to get that close to me. It became a safe haven. Basically speaking, being obese worked for me—until it stopped working. It worked until I got sick and tired of being sick and tired all of the time. It worked until I spent over 70 days in the hospital the year before my surgery. It worked until I decided I wanted to actually live, not just exist, until I wanted to thrive, not just survive.

I didn't tell anybody about the abuse for years. (I tried to tell someone one time, and that ended badly. Is it any wonder I never tried to tell anyone again?)

In 1991, my ex-husband was caught molesting one of our daughters. Because of my history I got them into therapy as soon as humanly possible. It was then that I began to address my own issues. I had basically stuffed it all down and when my children were abused it was as if someone took dynamite to the dam. We were all in therapy for about a year. About five years after that, I did another year of therapy to help me deal with the abuse from my mother. And before I had my surgery, I had another six months of therapy—it was then that I began to connect all the dots with the abuse and the obesity. I knew I had to get down to the bottom of my issue, or having the surgery would just be a colossal waste of time and money. I read hundreds of blogs before I decided to have my surgery.

I wanted to know the good, the bad, and the ugly. In all the blogs I read there were two things that jumped out at me when it came to long-term success: 1) A positive attitude—those who were successful 5, 7, 10-plus years out didn't focus on what they were losing or giving up. Their focus was on what they were gaining—a new life, health, doing things they wanted to do and couldn't do before, and 2) They all got therapy, either before or after surgery. They dealt with the issues behind the obesity. I have come to the conclusion that obesity is not so much a disease but a symptom of 'dis-ease.' It really is not what you are eating was much as it is what it is that is eating you."

What powerful, emotional, courageous contributions. The message in the preceding paragraphs is brilliant, insightful, and accurate. The preceding paragraph is worth writing on a note card for yourself and carrying with you. Read it frequently and heed the advice provided by one of your peers, who noted she learned about this from numerous others. Successful others. No point arguing with success.

I sure do love it when those words come from the people who have been down the road. So much more credible than when the psychologist says them! Sincere thanks to those who shared this very personal information for the benefit of others. One of the main reasons I wanted to write this book using the experiences of others and sending the message through their words, is because hearing that "therapy helps" coming from those who have benefit-ted from it *does* have more impact than a therapist recommending you go to counseling!

Abuse affects people on every level of their being. It usually takes the help of a trained professional to help a person move through the pain and damage that result from childhood abuse. Please get this professional help for yourself if you endured any sort of abuse in your childhood. Saying, "I've dealt with that," or "It happened so long ago," or "I'm an adult now," or "It's all in the past so what's the point of talking about it now," or "I've forgiven the abuser so why bring it up again?" does not mean you have truly worked through the pain. It follows you around, nipping at your heels like an obnoxious puppy on speed! It wants you to really deal with it! Turn around and face the past. Let yourself feel the feel-ings you felt at the time you were abused. Tell a professional how you felt at that time. Express your sadness, anger, grief, rage, fear, and whatever else you felt at the time of the abuse, in a safe envi-ronment with a professional. *Then* you can move on and not have the need to use food or other chemicals/behaviors to try to outrun or numb the pain.

Some days I wonder if almost everyone has experienced sexual abuse and then I remember I am a therapist and so I hear about it every day! Unfortunately, the number of children who are sexually abused is staggering. I don't want you to think, however, that it takes place in every household. In healthy families, sexual abuse does not occur. One of the reasons that sexual abuse so often goes unreported to officials by adults who are made aware of the abuse, is because the abuser is "my cousin," "my grandpa," "my aunt," "my brother-in-law," or some close family friend. People cover it up to prevent scandals and embarrassment. If I asked someone, "Would you willingly or knowingly contribute to a child being sexually abused?" they are usually mortified, get angry with me, and insist they would never do such a thing. When I inform them that, by not turning the perpetrator in to the authorities they are, in effect, willingly and (at least subconsciously) knowingly contributing to a child being molested. *How*? Because the statistics clearly point out that a child molester (be it your brother, niece, father, granny, or next-door neighbor) has numerous victims. *Numerous.* By "letting it go," or "sweeping it under the rug," or "turning a blind eye" if you are aware of someone molesting a child, you are, at the very least, failing to prevent the abuse from happening to other children. Will turning a person in to the authorities create some drama? Most likely. But who is responsible for that? The person reporting the crime, or the person who committed the crime? Please be courageous and report child molesters so other children are not harmed.

This next story is full of agonizing pain. The contributor bravely shares her immense grief with us. She notes how food turned to excess weight, which she hoped would bury her sadness, fear, pain, and shame. After she had weight loss surgery and was no longer able to use food in the way she had in the past, by trying to avoid her pain, she turned to alcohol in the hope that it would ameliorate her anguish. It did not. And her weight increased at the same time.

She did not state whether or not she has gone for therapy. My hope is that she has or will. She plans to work as a counselor to children as a way to help them through the kinds of horrible experiences she suffered. A great way to give back—as long as she has thoroughly worked through her issues in therapy! Please know—if you want to help others, *you have to have done your own work first!*

"My story starts out as a sad one. I am 36 years old. I am divorced and have no living children. As a child, I was sexually abused by five men in my family. It started at a young age and continued into my teenage years. I remember telling my friends in kindergarten that because their daddies did not 'touch' them, that their daddies didn't love them. I was the only one who was loved. I was seven years old when my parents divorced. At the age of 12, as the incest continued, I found myself pregnant. I DID NOT have a choice; I was COMPLETELY forced to have an abortion. From personal experience, I know how it feels to be violated, lonely, used, dirty, dead (inside), hurt, and filled with pain.

A girl often covers for the abuser because she is afraid of losing the person that she is led to believe is the ONLY person who really 'loves' her. She may be told that if she tells anyone, either no one will believe her or that she is a bad girl. I was made to believe that I could only be loved through sex. I was afraid of losing my father's love and I was led to believe that he loved me and that if I ever told anyone, no one would believe me. I felt insecure and had no one to comfort me. I had no one to protect me. ALL I wanted was to be loved.

I was told that I was doing the right thing by having an abortion because a baby should not come into the world if it was the product of incest or rape. I wasn't told that it would feel like a part of me was being 'sucked' out of my body—like my whole entire soul was being taken from me! I am not sure that my father knew what was going to happen at the abortion clinic. I was six-and-a-half weeks along and just couldn't even fathom a teen pregnancy which was the product of incest and rape. I experienced depression, sadness, guilt, anger, hurt, and pain after the abortion.

The abuse did not end there, and at the age of 15, I ended up pregnant again. Again I had another abortion, against my choice. I ended up contracting HPV when I was 10 or 11. The HPV became very severe. The physical disease stole my body. Also, from the time I was a small child, I was physically abused by my mother and stepfather. Sexual abuse from my father and psychological abuse from my mother, father, stepfather, and stepmother. My relationships with these people are not good at all. As a teenager and later in my adult life, I would get into relationships where sex was primary. I tried to search for love through sex.

At the age of 19, I got married. We were pregnant shortly thereafter. My marriage was on the rocks and I ended up having a miscarriage at nine weeks. I had developed high blood pressure. My life was sad and miserable. Then I got pregnant again, and three days after my twentieth birthday, I found out that we were being blessed with twins. Two weeks after that, we found out that they were both girls. I had a late second-trimester miscarriage/stillbirth. At this time, I had to deliver and have a D & C. From that surgery, I learned that I had endometriosis and polycystic ovarian syndrome (PCOS). Remarkably, I became pregnant again, and at eight weeks, I had yet another miscarriage. Two months later, I again suffered another miscarriage. By this time, I couldn't handle the physical and emotional abuse anymore and found out when I was getting ready to leave my ex-husband, that he was a homosexual. I actually walked in on him having sex with his lover. I had to leave because I thought that I would have hurt him.

I enrolled in nursing school in August of 1998. I met a guy who was in one of my classes, and found him easy to talk to and be with. So we got together. Ten months later I was pregnant and found out that I was again going to have twins—a boy and a girl. (Twins run in my family.) The father split. At the time, I was taking both my anatomy and physiology classes. I had severe morning sickness—all day long.

I quit school in October because the chemicals used in the labs made me sick. When I quit, I left town because I was ashamed. I fled to a big city. Two months later, my family talked me into coming home. On January 16, 1999, I had my baby shower. I received EVERYTHING! I became hypertensive again. I went in for my routine sonogram. My babies' heartbeats had stopped. I had no warning. That morning they were playful and kicking and within a few hours, nothing. I was eight months along and had to be induced. I was told because of my lack of a healthy weight gain, that I starved the babies to death. I couldn't keep anything down throughout my pregnancy. However, I was blamed and I still live with the guilt. Recently, I got out the death certificates and on my son's, it said that it was a cord accident.

After my first marriage and divorce, I had started gaining weight but I didn't see it. My family did, but there really was not any intervention. Just diets and Slim-Fast—no encouragement. As a child, I was sickly and thin. I miss 'thin' days!

Several months later, I met my husband. I got pregnant and again had another miscarriage at 11 weeks and 4 days on March 17, 2000. I went to a new doctor, who started me on some medications. Again, I became pregnant and again lost the baby.

At this point, I decided that I needed to see a specialist—a reproductive endocrinologist. That is when I learned that I have type 2 diabetes. I ended up needing to have a hysterectomy. Many pregnancies and no children.

In 2001, my husband and I separated, and in 2002, I finally made a motion for the judge to grant me a divorce. My husband was never supportive of me through any of my pain, especially when my babies' due dates and death dates came along.

In July 2004, I had gastric bypass surgery and as of now, March 2012, I have lost over 300 pounds. That weight I gained over all the years was like a cover for me. I didn't want to feel the pain of the abortions any longer. I have been denied plastic surgery two different times. I need to have this skin removed so that I can become healthier. Because of a job change, I no longer have insurance. So here I am with no husband, no children, and am so into my work that I have no time for myself. I did graduate from college in 2006. I just wish that I could really truly be happy—way down deep in my heart.

In 2008, I went through sexual harassment case at my workplace. It brought up ALL the memories of my past abuse. I could not handle the memories and therefore started drinking alcohol. When I started drinking, it was just random. Then I realized that the alcohol really numbed my pain. Well, the punch line here is that somehow I managed to let the drinking get out of hand. I got to where the emotional pain and memories became so bad, that I began drinking 30 cans of beer in four to five days.

I am a nurse, and I know the medical definition of an alcoholic. I didn't fit the picture. All I was trying to do was numb my pain. I would drink 'light' beer because I thought that it would not put the weight on me. Guess what? The beer put 40 pounds back on me. I began feeling like a failure because I misused the 'tool' of my surgery. Well, I am still struggling but I am working hard to get things right again.

I am currently pursuing my B.A. in psychology and planning on obtaining a double master's in child psychology and art therapy with a minor in nutrition. I do not want children to go through what I went through. If I can help stop the abuse and the increasing problem of obesity, then I will do what it takes to get there.

My grief for all my children is beyond degree, especially what I felt when I was forced into the two abortions. I finally understand and am able to cope with how the abortions affected me spiritually. I know that God understands the emotional pain that I have and I know that HE loves me. I just wish that those two abortions had never happened. I felt my miscarriages and still-births have a direct link with my abortions. That somehow I am being punished. I did name my children. Their names are Peyton Elizabeth, Sean Patrick, Matthew Luke, Dream Marie and Destiny Ann (twins), Isaiah Joel, Gabriella Faith, Joel Pate and Abagail Grace (twins), Madison Hope, Morgan Elisa, Whisper Faith, Haven Olivia, Kelsey Elise, and Gracie Elizabeth."

Many thanks to her for sharing the immense pain she has endured throughout her life. And greater thanks that she shared how she has chosen to help herself heal with the assistance of weight loss surgery. Losing weight and no longer drinking will allow her to continue to deal directly with the pain of her losses. Living sober at a healthy weight will also allow her to fully enjoy the benefits of living a healthy lifestyle.

Other forms of abuse also result in battered self-esteem. Emotional eating can be linked with verbal, emotional, and physical abuse, as noted by the following contributors:

"The abuse I suffered came in the form of verbal and emotional abuse from my dad. I don't think he ever realized it, quite honestly. And I was always afraid of my dad, so there was no way I'd ever tell him. To this day, I don't think he realizes it. To this day, I don't talk a whole lot with him. His teasing had a lot to do with my self-esteem, which led to my weight problems. I was called 'Porky' and teased from elementary school on up into high school.

I don't recall eating for comfort way back when I was in elementary school. I didn't start the emotional eating until high school. By then I lived with my mom, and it was the teasing from kids at school that got to me the most. Back when I was young, the only person who knew about my dad's teasing was my mom. I didn't really talk about it at all because I feared my dad. Eventually I came to believe I was no good anyway, so what was there to tell?

When my dad learned that I was getting weight loss surgery, I think that was the first time he'd ever stated he was proud of me. And after I was home from the hospital, he even brought flowers to my house. I was in complete shock. My mom passed away in 2006 due to morbid obesity–related issues. So she has no idea I've taken the surgical route.

After I had my own kids and gained even more weight, I did enter counseling. The treatment from my dad really affected me as an adult. I think I was about 24 or so when I first sought counseling. I continued to gain weight over the years and got to a high of 403 pounds. It was October of 2009 when I began the surgical process. I received the vertical sleeve gastrectomy on December 15, 2009. I've since lost 150 pounds and am still working on losing. I have another 85 pounds or so until I'm at my personal goal."

"I was spanked as a child. It felt as if I was spanked more than anyone else. My dad would take off his belt and pretend to spank my sister, but I would actually get spanked. My grandfather sometimes put his hand on my breast when we were tucked into bed. I always felt that was wrong, but unless I could sleep on my stomach, he always did it. I never talked to anyone about being abused."

"I was never abused until I encountered emotional abuse in Chicago. My ex-boyfriend was very obsessed with weight and would continue to make comments that really scared me pretty badly. We have since connected, and I now understand that his comments were not directed necessarily towards me, but were related to his own concerns about weight. I ate because I loved food. I loved going out to eat, having someone else prepare the meals, serve them to me, and then clean up. All I had to do was pay. And, boy, did I pay. I spent thousands of dollars in dining out every year."

"I was beaten with a belt by both of my parents, but my mother would lose it and really beat me. I remember one time when I guess I was being loud, (though I didn't think so) and my father was sleeping, she dragged me outside and threw me against a tree and started choking me, telling me to shut up and that if I woke my father up she was going to kill me. . . . I honestly have no idea what it is that I was doing at the time, for her to react like that.

My mother and my ex-husband were both verbally and emotionally abusive. I used to say that I would have preferred for them to just beat me. Physical abuse—I can fight back against that; it's right there in your face . . . emotional abuse sneaks up on you. I did not even recognize that my ex was emotionally abusive until I was out of the situation. Hit me—and I will either hit you back or walk away. Emotional/verbal abuse is insidious. And so much harder to defend against. And the longer it goes on, the less capable you are of defending yourself against it."

Abuse in childhood—always difficult to defend yourself against. For so many, as highlighted above, food was a way to protect oneself emotionally from the abuse. For a time, anyway. Please seek therapy and work through any abuse issues you have. It will be frightening to talk about your experiences, and you will feel emotions that have been buried for years. What is scary is that you will experience them in the present at the level of intensity you felt them in the past. In other words, even though you may be in your thirties, forties, or fifties, you will feel the fear as though you were 8 or 10 or whatever age you were when you experienced the abuse.

I personally believe this is often what prevents so many people from sticking with therapy. People get afraid of their feelings! They have worked so hard for so long to stifle the feelings, yet in therapy, they are paying someone to put them through those emotions! Adults often misunderstand the feelings they experience in therapy. They don't realize why the feelings are so intense and so frightening. It is because, as noted above, you will feel them with the intensity at which you experienced them as a child, when you did not have the ability to soothe yourself and you did not have the ability to process the feelings like you would now, as an adult. These reminiscent childhood feelings make grownups feel extremely vulnerable and childlike and out of control—not something we adults enjoy! Be brave. Face your fear with the knowledge that you are no longer in those abusive situations and you never have to go there again. You are now safe, and you can handle the feelings. But you must allow them. Then you can work through what happened—by talking about what you remember, how you felt, what you needed, and how you coped. The outcome of this process? You are free from having to fight those feelings that have been trying to escape for . . . decades, perhaps! You can now, as a healthier adult, give yourself permission to make healthy choices when you experience fear, sadness, anger, and other emotions instead of turning to food.

Please give it a try. It helps, I promise.

The next contribution is from a woman who struggled tremendously with obesity in her adult life. She endured personal tragedy and medical problems of her own. She found the strength within herself and through the help of loved ones to get through the dark times. She chose to have weight loss surgery and is now enjoying an exciting new hobby but is sharing the gift of healthy living following weight loss with some of her siblings!

"My top weight was 250 pounds, and at 5'5" I was miserable. I'm a mother of three. My youngest, Rachel, died on July 19, 1992 from a Wilms tumor. I probably weighed about 140 pounds at that time. I couldn't seem to find my place in the family after being the primary caregiver of Rachel for the 21 months of her illness. Previously, I had been active with my children and had enjoyed them all very much. At the time of Rachel's death, Amanda had just turned 12, and Jimmy had just turned 14 years old.

I had not been there for them for almost two years during Rachel's treatment, so I lost two of the most crucial years of their lives. I didn't know who I was. Jesus was the glue that held me together, and I spent the next several years trying to figure out just what to do with myself. Food became my addiction.

I had spent almost two years making medical decisions and caring for a very special child. In the process, however, I had lost my way with the other two children. Thus began my addiction to food (mainly carbohydrates, in the form of sweetened condensed milk with a spoon—the whole can—or a batch of fudge that didn't quite work out, also with a spoon and also the whole batch. The 10 years after my child's death took me over the 200-pound mark, and I couldn't find my way back.

In 1997, I was working for a physician in Dillard, Georgia, and tried phentermine. I actually lost about 35 pounds that way, but I developed migraine headaches and had to discontinue the use of it. I started back to school in 1998 to become a licensed practical nurse and did fairly well during the two years of training. I maintained my weight around 160 pounds by rigorously studying and then through the work I loved. I began my nursing career on the oncology ward and moved to the rehab ward when I had to take a day job for the sake of my health.

In 2000, I underwent treatment for hepatitis C. In 2001 I was diagnosed with carcinoma of my right breast, which was treated via lumpectomy; I later returned to have marginal tissue removed. During this time my weight began to climb at an alarming rate. I literally ate my own life up, and with the weight gain I developed additional alarming health issues. I was diagnosed with sleep apnea shortly after the time my weight topped the 200-pound mark. I became unable to work in 2001, being declared totally disabled.

By 2009 I was miserable. I had six wonderful grandchildren, and I didn't have the energy to play with them the way I wanted to. I hated what I had done to myself. The thing that helped me the most at that time was watching the weight melt off of my baby sister, Daisy. It was awesome! I was with her during her weight loss surgery. I made enough sugar-free Jell-o for her to sit in. I made it so beautiful with ribbons of different colors and flavors in pretty little cups. I was there to encourage her every step along the way. And then, in 2009, when I weighed in at 245 pounds, she said, 'You know, you can do it, too, if you want.' It took me almost a year to jump through all of the insurance hoops before my own weight loss surgery actually took place.

I'll never forget the day my sister Shirley and I were making the drive for the WLS initial seminar in Augusta, Georgia, when we passed a vineyard near Sandersville, Georgia. We stopped to pick some scuppernongs on the way, and I lost my prescription glasses in the orchard. On the way back we stopped to look for my glasses, and we knocked on the back door of the Anne Brickhouse home where we saw the most awesome pine needle baskets I had ever seen in my life. Anne showed us all the lovely baskets she had made and I told her that I would love to learn the art of pine needle basketry. She told me she would love to pass it on to me, so we began a yearlong game of telephone tag. My friend and I ended up at her house on August 13 for our first basketry class. While we sat at Anne's kitchen table learning, I got the call from the surgery center to inform me that I was on the surgical schedule for September. I was elated. . . . It all came full circle at my friend Anne's house and since that time I've made an important decision. . . . If I must have an addiction, I think I'll be addicted to pine needle basketry! It really helps!

As of this week I weigh 175 pounds. I have gone from a size 20 down to a 14-16. I love playing with my grandchildren. This Christmas I traded my Monopoly game for a trampoline. I still have the game because I know it's going to rain sometimes, but I'm ready to shed that other 50 pounds with my grandchildren this summer.

And, oh! Those 'Gotta-Do-'Ems'! I cannot even express the gratitude I have for them and the information in *Eat It Up!* But it all had to start with a made-up mind. I just purposed in my heart that with the help of the Lord I would make this journey to a healthier me. I am well on my way, and soon another of our sisters will join Daisy and me on this wonderful journey of weight loss and better health. Who knows, maybe even more of our sisters will make this journey. I'm feeling so good and looking forward to feeling better."

She gave me goose-bumps! Few of us can allow ourselves to imagine the heartache of losing a child. The woman did survive, and now she, too, is choosing to thrive in her life. She is sharing a healthy lifestyle with siblings, and together, they are blazing trails to a healthier life for the rest of their siblings, their children, and their grandchildren! And this woman sought out a person she admired and asked for help in learning a satisfying and beautiful skill! How about that for choosing health and paving a healthy path for her loved ones to follow?!

"Food became my addiction," she notes early in her story. She concluded whimsically by stating, *"If I must have an addiction, I think I'll be addicted to pine needle basketry!"* Addiction to food is a serious problem for a percentage of the obese population. For these people in particular, the possibility of playing "Whack-a-Mole addiction" following weight loss surgery is very real.

CHAPTER SEVEN

Obesity and Addiction

Yes—I ended the last chapter talking about "Whack-a-Mole addiction." Let me explain via a few paragraphs from *Eat It Up!*:

"One of my favorite games at the fair has always been Whack-a-Mole. If you have never played it, you really should. In fact, maybe all people who are recovering from any sort of addiction should invest in a home-version game of Whack-a-Mole. It would be a great thing to do instead of eating, *and* it would also serve as a great way to release anger in a healthy way. Just whack away at those infuriating little moles as they pop out of their holes. I digress. . . .

Whack-a-Mole is a game that has a table-top-like surface with several holes in it. The player holds a mallet in her hand, ready to strike. The goal is to whack the head of a little mole that pops up randomly in one or another of the holes in the table top. The more moles you whack in a certain amount of time, the better you do. This game is the perfect analogy for switching addictions.

Let's say, conveniently, that you are a food addict. Your addiction to food is represented by one of the moles in the game—the "food addiction mole" now has its head above the table. Let's now say that you decide to have bariatric surgery, which means that you are going to whack that little mole's head, and he disappears underneath the table top. *If all you do to lose weight is have bariatric surgery and do not engage in any of the other 10 items on the list* (exercise, food diaries, portion control, etc.) *it won't be long before another little mole pops his head out of another hole on the Whack-a-Mole table top.* This mole may represent drinking: it's the "drinking mole." You are no longer eating in a destructive manner, but have substituted alcohol. You are now drinking to numb yourself from painful emotions the way you used to eat to numb emotions. Let's say that your family members mention that you are drinking too much. They are uncomfortable with that and are worried about you. You don't want to be an alcoholic, so you pick up that Whack-a-Mole mallet and whack that "drinking mole" back down underneath the table top. When yet another mole pops up, you are curious. What now? Well, if you still haven't figured out that you are using other things like you use food, "other moles" will continue to pop up.

This time it's the "spending mole." In no time you realize that you have maxed out your credit card. You look at that mole head above the table top and tell it that in no uncertain terms you are in control, and that he is not going to win this round. Two more maxed credit cards later, out comes the mallet, and away you go, whacking at that little "spending mole." Before you even put the mallet down, up pops a "gambling mole." This cycle will go on and on and on unless you have the courage to recognize that you are literally replacing one addiction with another. Whack-a-Mole addiction!

Thirty percent of bariatric patients switch addictions. Many others regain their weight because, instead of switching addictions, they return to their "drug of choice," food. Have you ever condemned a person who successfully completes an alcohol or drug treatment program but returns to drinking just days or weeks after returning home? How different is that than when you lost a lot of weight but regained it?

It's hard to change. Old thought patterns, feelings, and behaviors are literally worn into your brain like tire tracks in wet mud. Changing the old thoughts, feelings, and behaviors, along with the old bad habits, is hard. But it can be done. *It can be done.* You can change your negative thoughts about yourself to positive thoughts about yourself. You can change your negative, destructive behaviors into positive, life-affirming behaviors."

So—that describes "Whack-a-Mole Addiction!" Many obese people resist the idea that food can be an addictive substance or that eating can be an addictive behavior. In the last paragraph of the previous chapter, I stated, "Addiction to food is a serious problem for a percentage of the obese population." The key words being *"for a percentage."* Not everyone who drinks is an alcoholic. Similarly, not everyone who is obese is a food addict. But some people who drink are alcoholics and some people who are obese are food addicts. Again, let me make my life easier and reprint (with my own permission!) a few paragraphs from *Eat It Up!* on the topic of food addiction:

Food/Eating: An Addiction?

"Minds are like parachutes—they only function when open," noted professor Thomas Dewar. I ask you to keep your mind open as you read this section. The word *addiction* often scares or angers people. Don't slam the door to your mind shut but read with curiosity. Give yourself a point for each category that follows if you can say "Yes" to the main question or to at least one of the examples in each category (or if you have experienced another situation that exemplifies the main question for the category).

Category One:
I often eat large amounts of food or eat for long periods of time or frequently throughout the day. (Yes or No)
- I often eat more than I intend to. For example:
  - I have additional servings even if I'm no longer hungry.
  - I take larger servings than I plan to.

- ○ I eat even though I am not hungry.
- ○ I eat even though I finished a meal recently.
- ○ I eat at mealtime and frequently between meals.
- ○ I am a grazer.

Category Two:

I have a persistent desire to lose weight or have had several unsuccessful efforts to lose weight. (Yes or No)

- I have started many diets that I have not stuck with.
- I have lost weight on diets but have regained my weight.
- I regularly say (out loud or to myself) that I want to lose weight.
- I have referred to myself as a "yo-yo dieter."

Category Three:

I spend (or have spent) a great deal of time or effort in activities necessary to obtain food, to eat food, or to recover from its effects. (Yes or No)

- I have gone out in the middle of the night to get some food I simply had to have.
- I have purchased more than one meal at a restaurant or drive-through (maybe even asking for a second drink so the cashier thinks I am buying food for additional people), even though all of the food is for me.
- I have done things like drive around looking for the 'HOT' sign at the donut shop, indicating there were fresh, warm donuts available.
- I have snuck food so others don't know I am eating it.

Category Four:

Important social, occupational, or recreational activities are given up or reduced because of substance use. (Yes or No)

- I have made special dates (with myself) just to eat as much of my favorite food(s) as I wanted.

- I have stayed up at night after everyone has gone to bed just so I could be alone to eat.

- I have missed work or other responsibilities because I was sick from eating too much.

Category Five:

I have continued to eat (or have not lost weight) despite knowing I have a persistent physical problem that is likely to have been caused or exacerbated by my weight. (Yes or No)

- I have one or more physical problems caused by, or made worse, by my weight:

  ○ High blood pressure.

  ○ High cholesterol.

  ○ Diabetes.

  ○ Knee or joint pain.

  ○ Sleep apnea.

  ○ Numerous others.

Category Six:

I need an increased amount of food to feel full or to achieve whatever the desired effect of food is OR in spite of eating the same amount of food as usual, it no longer satisfies me in the same way it used to.

- Sometimes I keep eating even though I am full because I am trying to feel better in some way.

- Food doesn't make me feel better anymore like it used to.

Category Seven:

I feel like I go through withdrawal if I am not able to eat when I want to, whether I am hungry or not, OR I use another substance (cigarettes, alcohol) or engage in another behavior (shopping, gambling) to deal with my feelings.

Add It Up

If you said yes to the main question (or to any of the examples in each category) for at least three of the categories, then you meet the criteria for substance dependence as described in the Diagnostic and Statistical Manual (IV), published by the American Psychiatric Association. The DSM defines addiction as "a maladaptive pattern of substance use leading to clinically significant impairment or distress, as manifested by three (or more)" of the criteria described in the categories above.

An ADDICT?

People don't like to be referred to as an "addict." Sounds so negative, doesn't it? The word "addict" has always had such a connotation. People tend to think of an "addict" as a gutter drunk, a homeless heroin junkie, a "crack head" prostitute. Or at least that's how it was in the past. Sadly, for many people, the word "addict" still brings to mind the picture of a less-than-desirable human being. The reality is, however, that addicts come in the form of janitors, cardiologists, psychologists, garbage collectors, stay-at-home moms, English teachers, judges, accountants, nurses, cashiers, and every other profession. All races, the old and the young, male and female; anyone can be an addict.

Addicts are people whose use of a chemical (including alcohol) or whose behavior (eating, gambling) has caused problems for them—in relationships, work, school, or in other areas of responsibility. Some would say that addiction is present when a substance or behavior has "gotten out of control." This definition often causes too many problems, as far as I'm concerned, as most addicts love to swear they can "control" their use or behavior. For simplicity's sake, therefore, let's put aside the "control" aspect of addiction for a moment and go with the idea that an addiction is present when the substance or behavior has caused problems for a person. I'm not talking problem, as in one incident, such as sitting on the boss's lap after drinking too much (although that can't be good). I'm not talking about spending too much money on a wardrobe after you get your first professional job. I'm not talking about eating so much on Thanksgiving that you aren't able to play football with your kids or you'll throw up (even though they'll probably be upset with you).

I'm talking about PROBLEMS. You know, like getting a DUI the week after you sat on the boss's lap, which it turns out, happened two weeks after you and your spouse had a big fight about how your behavior changes around men after you drink too much. I'm talking about having spent too much money on a new wardrobe after you have maxed out three credit cards, and after you told your spouse you had already cut up the credit cards. I'm talking about overeating on Thanksgiving and continuing to overeat daily while gaining more and more weight after your doctor tells you that you are on the verge of developing type 2 diabetes, after he told you two months ago that you had developed high blood pressure, which happened after he already told you that your cholesterol was dangerously high. Problems that continue after you are already aware that the substance or behavior has caused problems. Those kinds of problems indicate addiction.

Approximately 30 out of every 100 people who have bariatric surgery "switch addictions." Some postsurgical people start drinking and continue drinking even when serious problems arise as a result. Some start spending money irresponsibly even after financial problems arise. Some start having sex with almost anyone, which is problematic for a variety of health reasons.

The following story is from a contributor who bravely shares her struggles with various forms of addiction: relationships, drugs, and the rollercoaster of weight loss and regain. She has clearly learned a tremendous amount about life, love, and what brings her true happiness. She has acknowledged and accepted that she is an emotional eater. Not turning to food for comfort remains a struggle in her life, but she is working hard to maintain healthy new habits. This woman has a lifetime of fighting through tough times. By learning positive coping strategies, she will find it easier and easier to walk away from unhealthy food and other unhealthy ways of trying to ease emotional pain.

This Is an Addiction story . . .
Weight Loss Surgery Story—What Led to My Obesity and My Breaking Point

"I would give anything to have a 'do-over' in this life. To begin again, knowing what I know now.

My story of my destination to obesity begins at the age of 17. I never planned on getting pregnant at such a young age, but I thought since I was so . . . 'in love' . . . oh, well. Now I'll be a mom, too. I can get married and move out of the house. I now realize that was the best place to be. Becoming an adult and living on my own sounded so fun, and I would have no one to answer to, right?

So there I was— pregnant at 17 with no knowledge of how to take care of myself, let alone a husband a child—and I had to work to help pay rent! Wait, this isn't at all as fun as I thought it was going to be. Food. Yes, my friend. The one thing I did have control of. Or did it really have the control? For a while, I felt good with my new love, and even though we didn't have a lot of money, food was cheap at McDonald's. Because I was damned with morning sickness, nothing felt better than going to the drive-through every morning and getting a couple orders of salty French fries. . . . I gobbled them down on the way to work, and by the time I got there, I felt so much better. It's no surprise in my nine months of being pregnant that I gained a whopping 87 pounds!

By the time I gave birth to the most beautiful gift I have ever received, I was 240 pounds and was only 17 years old. From then on I would never be anything but a fat mom. Years passed by me, so fast I honestly don't remember too much until I was 22. That was when I started wondering if I was really in love with this man who hadn't really done anything wrong. I just woke up one morning and changed my mind. I wanted more. I wanted to be a real person, and I wanted to do something. I wanted to be noticed! This is where my 30 years of dieting began.

I think the first diet gimmick I heard about was diet pills. I went to a doctor, who had a little shop in a little strip mall. He gave me some test, and before he could possibly have gotten any results back, he handed me a bunch of pretty pills. Let's just say they became my 'new love' for the time being. I was on these pills for so long, my mom actually had an intervention with me so I could get off them. I lost so much weight. I weighed 122 pounds. At 5'8" that was terrifying! But I needed those dolls! I was freaking hooked. My hubby forbade me to go back on them. At my new, slender weight, I was now a new person. I was sexy, I was young, and I didn't need someone making rules for me. Especially someone who was now drinking and staying out late all the time. I knew it was because we had fallen out of love with each other. All I knew was that I wanted my pills to make me not eat. To keep me thin!!

Needless to say, my marriage was not at a healthy stage, so we decided to separate, just to see if we really wanted to be together. We never did get back together, but the beautiful thing about him and me, that I have always been so proud of, is that we have remained friends. No fighting, no jealousy, no threats. We probably should have always been just that. Good friends.

My daughter always had the best of both of us. At least during her childhood.

Well, there I was, finally free, not having to answer to anyone. I had a nice home, and two wonderful kids. Oops! I forgot to mention, I was also raising my seven-year-old nephew. My sister was unable to raise him by herself. She had MS by the time he was a year old and there [were] a lot of drugs and fighting, so I took him. I wanted him to feel like he was part of a good home. Yeah, well I really believed my children were in a happy home. I think I should have been awarded the Oscar because they only saw a happy, thin Mom. I was working two jobs!! I owned my own beauty shop, and worked in a steakhouse/bar at night.

I then started gaining back the weight pretty rapidly. I was working a lot of hours, and thank goodness I met 'Annie,' a fellow waitress. She showed me how to work the hours I was working, have a good time doing it, and lose some weight too. She introduced me to cocaine.

My world was complete, I was making great money, working day and night, having fun, and getting skinny. Dang, I had it made. But wait, I had two kids at home. Granted, I never left them alone; they always had everything they wanted. They were happy. But I wasn't.

This wasn't me. This wasn't fun. I wanted a relationship. In walked a new man—who would soon be the worst nightmare of my life. I can't even speak his name, so we will call him, HIM. To make a long story short, he moved in with me and controlled every minute of my life. I don't know what happened to me. I think I was possibly brainwashed because I became someone I didn't even know. I was never someone who took grief from anyone, but I truly feared for my life in the nine months I was with HIM. Let's just say that after too many beatings to count, he went to jail, and I lost all sense of self-worth. Here I was, getting fatter and fatter. Again.

After that, if you can believe it, I actually remarried, to someone I thought would help me feel better about myself. Guess what—he was an alcoholic. Enough said. That marriage surprisingly lasted 10 years. During that time of my life I think I lost and gained back the same 100 pounds three times. I again believe I was blessed to get out of that relationship alive.

At this point, I was now 44 years old and moving back in with my mom. Need I say more? Two strong-willed women living in the same house. All I can say is—she was always there for me.

Hold on to your hats, folks. I was divorced a little over one year, and I met a new man. Now I know what you're thinking: NOT AGAIN! I weighed 260 pounds at the time and this guy liked me? I didn't get it. I was then on the list to start Optifast. I was so excited about the prospect of losing this weight for the final time. Eight months later, after not putting a bite in my mouth, except the five shakes a day, I was now thin again, for my wedding. Okay, I guess you have the right to roll your eyes at me, but this one will be forever. We had been married about four years, and he truly was the man of my dreams. We talked. There was no yelling and no fighting, and all was wonderful in Paradise.

In the meantime, my precious Mom was battling with her own demons. She started seeing things, getting lost, and became too scared to be left alone. I knew the signs; you see, my father had dementia when he died. What were the odds of both of my parents being afflicted with this?

My husband sat me down one evening and suggested we move in with Mom so she could have company and not be afraid. I immediately agreed. As I said before, she was always there for me. My husband built me another beauty shop at my mom's house, and I was able to be there all the time. ALL the time. OMG! I love my mother, more than anyone in the entire world, but I didn't know how to take care of someone who was deteriorating so quickly, right before my eyes. In the five years we were with her, I gained back all of my weight, plus.

I guess you can say for absolute sure, I am a stress eater. And I had never in my life felt so stressed. There were times I thought I was going to have a mental breakdown. When my mother got to the point that she became violent, I was becoming a little afraid I might wake up dead. Truly, people, I had to call EMTs out to treat me as a result of her lashing out. This was no longer my precious Momma. She was sick, and I could no longer care for her. She is now in a wonderful nursing home. They take exceptional care of her, and she is beyond the angry stage. In fact, we are just waiting for her to go home to the Lord.

I had my RNY gastric bypass five months after she was placed into care, September 15, 2008. I lost 85 pounds, and although I have not reached my goal, I am happy. My husband and I just celebrated our eleventh anniversary. We are still in love. We have plans to move to Hawaii, and really live in Paradise. I am still struggling with keeping the weight off.

But I am happy."

This woman's story is like so many others' stories. So often we look for external ways to battle our internal demons. Neither diet pills nor cocaine solved anything for her, nor do they for anyone. They just keep us removed from reality. Sadly, they also keep us emotionally removed from our children and others we love. One bad relationship after another didn't help heal any of her internal pain, and never will. Working so many hours that we remain emotionally distant from ourselves doesn't fix anything, either. With all of these things—drugs, bad relationships, excessive working—all we lose are valuable years during which our kids grow up or we grow more unhappy. Fortunately, with time and learning from her mistakes, this woman has been able to find the kind of love we all want. In turn, she is demonstrating increased self-love. Having weight loss surgery is an example of how she showed she believes that she matters. She matters enough to get help for her obesity. Continual work at keeping the weight off further shows her commitment to and love of self. This in turn, will make that loving relationship even more joyful!

The following woman's story is one that does not speak of addiction and yet, she honestly acknowledges that she used food, and now uses alcohol, to try to fill the hole in her soul. She has tremendous insight and has ultimately made positive choices for herself. Her ability and willingness to identify that she used food as a friend and is now "flirting" with alcohol abuse/addiction, reflects her conscious awareness of what she needs to work on. The fact that she has been, and remains in therapy, indicates she continues to want a healthy lifestyle. Awareness is always the first step in change. And past choices are often a good predictor of future choices. Things bode well for this woman!

> "I was not a heavy child. In fact, I was often told I was 'skinny' by friends and family. I did not start gaining weight until I was over 30, but I can tell you how the early messages I received contributed to my ultimate obesity. It was great to be lauded for my 'skinniness,' but there was not much substance for me behind that.
>
> My childhood was chaotic. My parents fought often and I felt unwanted from an early age. I was the youngest of four children. First there were two girls and then my brother. I was three-and-a-half years younger than him. He wanted a baby brother in the worst possible way, as his sisters tormented him. In his disappointment, he tormented me. My father was volatile and unpredictable. My mother struggled to appear 'normal,' as she suffered from extreme anxiety. The only thing she could be was

self-centered, and she passed her anxiety on to me, the 'sweet one.' My dad fluctuated between episodes of over-indulgence and abusive rage. My mother was consumed by appearances and what the neighbors might think. As I grew, I tried to be the mediator in their marriage. I played the role of the 'good one.' Ultimately, I rebelled and ran off at a young age with a much older man who only exploited me.

When I returned home, crippled by anxiety in my early twenties, my parents' marriage was at the breaking point. My mother would run into my room at night screaming, 'He hit me!' while my father proclaimed that he had no choice. I spent many hours analyzing my life with my dad, while he seemed to understand. But ultimately, the truth was revealed. He had been having a 20-year affair, and our once well-to-do family was headed for bankruptcy. He blamed everyone but himself. My acting out, he claimed, was a big cause of his undoing. He felt that all of his children were 'cold, cruel, and contemptible.' This was expressed during calls at 2:00 a.m., during which he said he was sorry for having children. Ultimately, he proclaimed the same words in a courtroom, where he attempted to sue all of his offspring for 'ingratitude,' if you can believe this is even possible. My dad ultimately divorced my mother and his children during my late twenties and early thirties. He married the woman with whom he had been having his affair and decided that all of his children (and somehow, I thought, especially me) had been the cause of all his problems. He is still not a part of my life.

Meanwhile, during this chaos, my mother was able to think of little but her own struggles. The way she makes herself feel better is by her own good appearance. My mother receives many accolades for appearing younger than her age, and she is always dressed impeccably. Simultaneously, she was consumed by shame, embarrassment, and anxiety. She had, and still has, a habit of examining me through the lower half of her bifocals and making some comment about my appearance.

My own anxiety and distress kept me thin for many years. I ended up marrying a man who seemed calm and compassionate. He was both of these things but was also frustrating and withholding. Eventually, I gained some control over my anxiety, but my depression was always knocking at the door. Once the anxiety was better controlled with therapy and medication, my appetite grew. At first, it felt like a sign of health. But I was still in a frustrating marriage and feeling that I was responsible for almost anything that went wrong. As my frustration grew, so did my size. Therapy and antidepressants helped to tame my demons, but I think the meds also increased my appetite.

Eleven years later my husband and I divorced. I felt guilty (mostly about our five-year-old son), responsible for the failure of the marriage, worthless, and I was fat! As I grew larger, I could see my mother's shame. She often offered advice and comments about the best ways to diet and control my weight. As you can imagine, I only felt anger and resentment. The more she monitored my eating, the more I wanted to eat. The more I ate, my inner critic screamed louder and louder. My weight became both my friend and my enemy. Of course I could not date . . . right? But I resented men for not seeing beyond my appearance. I saw in everyone's eyes what I expected . . . what I felt all my life . . . that I was not wanted or worthy. If there was a problem, it was most likely my fault. Why would anyone want someone like me? And if they expressed interest in me, I only wondered what was wrong with them.

So, as time ticked on, my weight hung on. I felt like my appetite was increasingly out of control with little hope that I would ever find a desirable partner. I had been in therapy for many years and continued my quest for self-exploration. I felt that I worked through many of the issues related to my divorce but was unable to fill the hole that seemed to reside in my gut. As I tried to fill the hole with food, satisfaction was always outside my reach. As all overweight people do, I gained and lost weight, but there was a hungry monster inside that could not be tamed. Although I had not yet suffered severe health consequences, I could feel the toll my weight was taking on my body and soul. I wanted to feel more desirable. Maybe the critics (the ones in my mind and the ones outside of me) could be silenced if I could do something about my appearance. The first step had to be weight loss, and the only hope for a more enduring solution seemed to be WLS. After some thought and research, I decided the vertical sleeve gastrectomy was my best option, and four years ago I had my surgery.

In the days following surgery I can honestly say that I mostly thought, 'What have I done to myself?' I felt pretty miserable and could not comfort myself with my old friend, food. But I kept reminding myself of the goal and hung in there with the knowledge that I would soon feel and look better. The pounds began melting off, and the accolades came. In the following months, I melted down and down until I felt like one hot mama! The compliments came pouring in, and I felt great! I exercised and ate right. I did activities that I wouldn't dare do before, like zip-lining over the jungle. I could cross my legs, tighten the airplane seatbelt, and go to the water park with my son. I had 'the girls' repositioned and whitened my teeth. I joined a dating service and started dating. Yay me!

Okay, but here's the rest of the truth. I still miss filling my old large belly with comfort food. I have gotten much more used to this and remind myself when I miss food that the benefits outweigh (get it?) the sacrifice. So, missing food is okay with me now—for the most part. However, somehow the weight loss did not miraculously cure my inner critic. It did not magically empower me, cure my depression, and fill that gnawing hole in my soul. It did not summon Prince Charming to my door. When a man now gives me sexual attention, I am flattered, but I must admit that I still feel that he doesn't see 'me,' and I still wonder, 'What is wrong with him?' Hmmm, go figure. I am now four years post-op and still without a male companion.

During the last year, I have discovered that drinking helps me to temporarily forget about that hole in my soul and it quiets my inner critic. So, the drinking has slowly increased, and I know I am flirting with another dangerous demon. When the WLS honeymoon ended, so did the exercise. Didn't I promise myself I wouldn't let this happen?! I have, so far, maintained a healthy weight, and I am grateful for all the benefits I enjoy that came from my weight loss, but clearly the war wages on."

The above stories are two examples of how people use food as one means of avoiding the pain of their past or the feelings accompanying one's present reality. Addiction, whether it is to food, to alcohol, to drugs, to relationships, or to any number of other things, always negatively interferes with relationships. Obesity, whether a person is addicted to food or not, also interferes with relationships. Think about the ways your obesity has, or does, interfere with your personal relationships. Take a good look at yourself and ask if you are playing "Whack-a-Mole" and using other substances or behaviors to try to keep you from dealing with issues in your life, past or present. Listen to others around you. They'll tell you, directly or indirectly, if they have concerns about your shopping/spending, drinking, use of recreational or prescription medications, use of the computer/Internet, or any other behavior you may be engaging in too frequently. If you are abusing other substances or engaging in a behavioral addiction, get help and do so immediately, before you end up with another whole set of problems to address!

Blogger Cari De La Cruz wrote about recovery from her own food addiction on her web page www.bariatricafterlife.com:

FOR OR AGAINST?

"This morning, when I awoke and committed to my 4th Day of Sobriety, I figured out that recovery from obesity is a choice, and one that I must make clearly and resolutely every, single day.

So, I began my new mantra: Today, I choose life. I choose to be healthy. I choose to control what I put in my mouth. I choose to give power only to food that will bring me closer to recovery.

It would have been very easy to say: Today, I will NOT eat things that I shouldn't eat. I will NOT eat Fruit Loops, or that Carrot Zucchini bread. I will NOT overdo it. I will NOT eat the wrong things. I will NOT give into my addiction. I will NOT binge.

In other words, I could choose to make a list of things I will NOT do—OR, I can make statements about what I WILL (and have the power to) do.

Sidebar: Oh my gosh! It just hit me that this concept of standing 'for' something is a lot like our Constitution. The Constitution doesn't GIVE us power as individuals; it simply states the God-given power that we ALREADY HAVE. Hmmm . . . interesting. I need to go FOR or AGAINST? There is a difference between fighting AGAINST something and standing FOR something. Neither is particularly wrong, but each carries with it a different source of power; a different attitude; a different way of thinking and being.

- I can fight against negativity in my workplace, or I can stand for having a good attitude in all that I do.

- I can fight against negativity in my home, or I stand for a positive spirit.

- I can fight against negativity online, or I can stand for upbeat, hopeful truth.

There is NOTHING WRONG with fighting for what you believe; fighting for a cause; fighting for the truth. Many choose to fight against something, because it feels good to belong to a bigger, more powerful cause; it feels productive and purposeful; it feels better than standing ALONE.

Sometimes, people choose the fight, the battle, or the war, INSTEAD OF peace, because they want to change people, or bring them to their side; they want others to join their team, and they want to feel powerful. After all, there's great power in numbers, it's good to belong, and there is a place and purpose for fighting for what you believe. It is good to make clear choices on where you stand.

But, in this context—the subject of ADDICTION—I have begun to ask myself this question: Do I want to fight with an army of thousands or stand as an army of one?

I know that there are millions of people fighting against their addictions. I would not be alone in my battle. But fighting AGAINST something takes more energy than STANDING FOR something, and I believe that fighting AGAINST my addiction would be harder than standing FOR recovery.

I guess you could say that I have chosen to stand alone, BUT I am encouraging others to stand with me—if they want. The truth is, I can no more fight another's battle than they can win mine, but I can champion and support them in standing for what's right.

So, that's where I am in my Bariatric After Life™: I am not fighting AGAINST my addiction; I am choosing to stand FOR sobriety. Are you standing for something? Are you fighting against something? Are you doing both or neither?"

CHAPTER EIGHT

Living Life after Weight Loss Surgery

Throughout this book, you've read some awesome blog posts by Cari De La Cruz. You've also read a term she has coined, a term she uses to refer to life after bariatric surgery. She calls it the "Bariatric After Life." I asked her to write a few paragraphs about how she came up with that terminology, since living life after weight loss surgery, or living the Bariatric After Life, is what this chapter is about. Here's what she said:

> "I never thought of myself as a writer, mostly because I didn't enjoy it, but also because I didn't believe I was very good at it. But I have learned that what we *believe* to be true about ourselves is not always *actually* true . . . which, as it turns out, explains both *how* and *why* I ultimately became a blogger, vlogger, and social media fixture.
>
> In my 'before life,' I knew I was a good speaker; I just didn't think I had anything good to say. So, while I could comfortably address a graduating audience of 5,000 people at my college commencement, I couldn't imagine what *else* I could talk about. Thanks to weight loss surgery, I found my answer: *I could talk, write, and share about graduation from obesity and commencement to recovery!*
>
> And that's exactly what I did. I began spreading the good news of life after bariatric surgery by launching *'Gastric Bypass Barbie'*—a blog and video channel about changes in my life,

changes in what I ate and did . . . and changes in shoes. That's right: *shoes!* Because life is serious enough without worrying about how to choose the right shoes.

Perhaps more than that, I wrote about how losing weight opened doors I never even knew existed . . . and the more I wrote, the more I learned that I was not alone in my thoughts. I learned that others suffered from the disease of obesity, wrestled the same demons and waged the same battles I did. Most importantly, I learned about addiction and recovery.

Over time, as I interacted with more and more post-ops, I began to see a disturbing trend. I watched as people tied their success to an arbitrary number on the BMI chart, a random weight on their scale, or a size on their jeans. In dismay, I watched as people declared that they would only be happy when they could bookend their 'before' picture with a victorious 'after' picture.

Sadly, many believe that a happy life comes down to a picture and a number—but life is more than just a single moment in a snapshot or on a scale. *Real* life is everything after the 'after' picture—the goal number, the surgery—the obesity.

Real life is what I live every day, and I call it the *Bariatric After Life*™—not because I died, but because I was given a second chance to live. Life after bariatric surgery should be a celebration of life after death; rebirth from failing health to good health, from sadness to joy, from sickness to recovery—and everything in between. The *Bariatric After Life* is the death of old ways and birth of healthy new behaviors and attitudes; it is living life on life's terms.

As you've probably guessed, I'm passionate about the subject of the *Bariatric After Life,* so it's nearly impossible to keep it to myself. Fortunately, that's what this book is all about: *Finding your voice, spreading the message of hope, health and recovery, and paying it forward.*

At the end of the day everyone has a message to share, and *everyone* can help *someone.* When you believe in yourself, the message speaks for itself."

And that explains the Bariatric After Life, which is a day-by-day endeavor that requires continuous effort. The following blog post by Cari makes that very clear:

UNVARNISHED TRUTH

WARNING: If you don't want to hear the truth,
stop reading this right now.

Living a healthy and successful bariatric after life doesn't just happen by accident. It takes tons of planning and preparation. Unfortunately, when many people "sign up" for the surgery, they focus more on what they read in the "marketing materials" and less on what living, breathing people tell them.

- Who wouldn't want to believe that surgery really is the "easy way out?"

- Who would knowingly sign up to have their insides completely rearranged and NOT know that their life-style would have to be permanently and radically altered—forever?

- Who could actually believe they'd be able to "eat what-ever they want" after surgery (just "less of it") and not gain weight?

- Who would subject themselves to all of this and NOT understand what it would take to succeed?

- Who would have bariatric surgery and NOT understand that success only happens when preparation meets opportunity?

How about MOST bariatric patients?

It never ceases to amaze me when I hear someone complain about having to measure their food, log their nutritional stats, pack ahead before leaving the house, or exercise regularly. I just want to say (in my best Dr. Phil voice), "How's that workin' out for ya?"

I mean, COME ON!

I didn't become Morbidly Obese by accident. I weighed 316 pounds because I didn't want to be accountable to myself. I didn't want to be burdened with measuring food, planning ahead, going to the gym, or eating healthy foods. That might sound like a bitter pill to swallow, but, in my Bariatric After Life, I've had to come to terms with some harsh and painful realities: I was entirely responsible for my obesity. Oh, sure, there were miti-gating factors and, like any "accident," I can try to blame my condition on a perfect storm of situations over which I can argue I had no control. But that wouldn't help me now, and it wouldn't change the past.

That's why I decided from day one post-surgery that I would do whatever it took to lose my weight and NEVER GO BACK.

Okay, so I didn't realize that would involve measuring my food. And I didn't know I'd be packing lunches and snacks every day for the rest of my life. And I wasn't aware that I'd have to carry an insulated lunch bag with protein. No one told me I'd be exercising 5+ days a week—at the ungodly hour of 5:30 a.m. I wouldn't believe that I'd be able to drink a protein shake for breakfast every day and not get bored with it. I had no idea I'd have to understand the difference between a complex carb and a simple carb. I wasn't prepared for the complete and utter change in my behaviors, attitudes and actions.

But . . . This is my life. It's what I do. And I love it.

The way I see it, you can either fight reality, or find a way to embrace it and thrive. I've chosen the latter, and the result shows. Oh, it's not easy, but it sure is rewarding.

So, to all of you out there who say you don't want to pack little mason jars and store them in the fridge. For those who say you hate protein shakes. For anyone who complains that they can't wait 5-10 minutes between bites, give up carbonated beverages, or never eat and drink at the same time again, I have one thing to say: No problem. But don't complain to me when the weight starts to creep back on and you can't figure out "why."

Harsh? Maybe. But, my dad always said, "Experience keeps a dear school, while a fool will have no other." In English? Learn from others' mistakes and then do the work. You'll never regret it. I promise.

—Cari De La Cruz (www.bariatricafterlife.com)

Recovering from Obesity

Obesity is a chronic disease. There is no cure. There is only maintenance. Sustaining weight loss *requires* daily maintenance. Getting the weight off, made easier with the tool of weight loss surgery, is truly only the *beginning*. Ask anyone who is two years or more out from their weight loss surgery. The *only* thing that weight loss surgery makes easier is the *initial* weight loss. From that point on, it requires tremendous effort and ongoing effort.

Chronic diseases like obesity remit; they are not cured. You will forever be in a state of recovering from obesity. You will never be "recovered." Recovering from obesity entails dealing with more than the physical changes resulting from surgery. The daily choices you face about what you eat, when you eat, how much you eat, and where you eat are part of your recovery process. If, when, and how you exercise are parts of your ongoing process of recovering from obesity. The thoughts you choose to focus on and the subsequent feelings and behaviors are part of your recovery from obesity. Recovery from obesity includes your daily behavioral choices, the quality of the thoughts that you choose to entertain, and whether or not you utilize a healthy support system to include professional counseling.

The following contribution tells the tale of initial weight loss followed by the reality of "normal" life exceptionally well:

The Day after the Big Game

(AKA: Being Normal)

"The confetti has stopped falling.
The crowds have cleared out of the stands.
The pep band is packing away their instruments.
There will be major headlines in tomorrow's papers!
But I stand here, at center court, sensing that the pinnacle of all the excitement has just been reached. I've just defeated an historic rival, and this has been my moment.
After this, there will only be an occasional line or two written in the newspaper about the day of the 'big game.'
Someone may stop me in the street every now and then to give me a big high five and a fond chuck to the ribs.
And rarely, conversations might come up where someone remembers this day and asks me to recount how it came about.
It wasn't supposed to be like this. I'm not sure what exactly it was supposed to be like, but this isn't it. How is it that a person

can do what seems to be a monumental task only to find one-self standing in silence? The cheers, the pats on the back, the gasps of delight, and the public congratulations were so prolific and so intoxicating while I was losing weight. Everyone seemed to have a kind or encouraging word to say, regardless of the situation. But as the newness of my achievement has worn off, those things have all but trickled to a stop. People have become accustomed to me as 'normal' sized. They see me walk down a street or into a room, and I'm 'just J.' I get a normal greeting with none of the additional delight that has been my experience for the past two years.

How can that be? I mean, I've just won the big game for the hometown team. I've just beaten an age-old rival. This is what they all wanted for me. I was obese for nearly 40 years. I've been 'normal' for less than one. I'm not used to normal. How in the world can they be?

The truth is that the task of being normal isn't over for me. I have to play in that same championship game every single day of my life in order to maintain my weight loss. To all concerned, I have reached maintenance weight. However, my disease of chronic morbid obesity is not cured. The disease is merely in remission. It doesn't go away just because my weight 'looks' normal. The surgical tool helps with the battle tremendously and even makes it winnable. But, it will never cure the obesity. I guess maintenance is not the sexy battle. A daily struggle to maintain a weight is not worthy of cheers or atta-boys. It doesn't make headlines, and unless I mention it, it doesn't even pop up on other people's radar screen. Come to think of it, it is an unseen battle much like those that are fought by many individu-als who are faced with a variety of chronic diseases.

My surprise at the silence associated with becoming a nor-mal-sized person has a history. There's a huge buildup to weight loss surgery; the research, the evaluation by the bariatric team, the medical tests, the decision to go ahead with the surgery, the pre-op weight loss, attending support groups, hearing the sto-ries, asking questions, breaking the news to friends and rela-tives, clearing the house of contraband, dealing with the pre-op bowel prep, and waking up before dawn on the day of surgery. While at the hospital, the patient is the center of attention. It is all new; it is all exciting. A new era has begun. There is hope that a solution to the chronic morbid obesity with all of its baggage has finally been found. There is also a companion tension that niggles, 'What if this doesn't work for ME?'

The first several months I think I was simply in amazement. I could not believe that it was even possible for weight to come off that fast. I was going through clothing sizes like nobody's business. I was trying not to shop too much, but it was WAY too much fun. I would tell myself that I was buying things that would fit for several months. HA! I just wanted to look better and better as the weight came off. Each time I saw a friend or a co-worker, especially if there had been an extended period of time between contacts, there were squeals of delight, looks of amazement, and requests for me to share my 'secret.' I also found that I was like a born-again bandster. I wanted to save every obese person in the world.

I became the center of attention on a regular basis, and all I had to do was walk in a room. I was melting into a rather attractive 40-something woman who already had a lot going for her before the weight loss ever happened. I loved turning heads. In the past, the only heads I turned were the ones that either turned away in disgust at my largeness or turned to look with a scowl at the enormity of my size. I felt like I was walking on air to get positive attention in relation to my physical appearance. It was a brand new experience for me.

There was this odd sense of power that came along with becoming attractive by society's standards. I am a tall woman with exceptionally long legs. So, as I became smaller and began to walk with my head up in a confident stride, heads turned; especially those that were of the male persuasion. I smiled and reveled in the ability to make a teensy bit of a wave wherever I went. Of course, being the dramatic performer that I am, I never just eased into a room. I made an entrance. Making the wave, no matter how slight, was intoxicating.

Feeling so powerful and accepted for the first time in my life made the daily work of becoming thinner and healthier extremely easy to deal with. There were immediate rewards. There was an instant sense of gratification. If I had a brief moment of fear or disappointment about my progress, all I had to do was to walk out my door and into anyplace where there were people in my small town. I would bump into someone who hadn't seen me in a while and get 'the squeal.' There. I've had my fix for the day.

I was not prepared for what would happen when the stadium

lights went dim and the crowds grew silent. Somehow I had unconsciously come to believe that being thinner would always be fun. I had the mistaken idea that thin girls were at the center of attention simply because they were thin. I know that I didn't believe that being thin would solve all of my life's problems, but I did have some deep-seated, unspoken belief that it would be just shy of fabulous.

It's not. It's just normal. Compared to the previous two years of my life, it's actually downright boring. The high that I have been living on is gone. The days of getting an instant adrenaline and endorphin fix through 'the squeal' are past. I'm sure that the dosage tapered gradually, but my awareness of its absence seems to be as if someone did an intervention and made me go cold turkey.

And I still have a battle to fight. I have to play the big game on a daily basis in order to keep the age-old rival of morbid obesity at bay. It's just that the battle is confounded by the fact that it occurs in an empty stadium. There's no confetti, no pep band, and no roaring crowds. I can ASK the cheerleaders to be there if I really need them. But I can't ask them to follow me around 24/7. I would wear them out. This means that one of the toughest parts of normal is that I have to battle my rival without an artificially elevated level of performance enhancing neurotransmitters.

Somehow the foe has to be held at bay for an intrinsic reason—and that reason can't be fear. Fear is an easy substitute for elevating those performance-enhancing lovelies that my brain creates. If I stay in a perpetual state of fear that my weight is going to come back, then fight or flight keeps the ol' adrenalin pumping. It's certainly not as fun as the atta-boys, but it works (at least temporarily). I'm not sure how to make the transition from stadiums full of cheering fans to a still, small voice inside of myself as the motivation to continue my daily, boring, mundane attempt to hold the line against a rival that will push back at the first opportunity.

It is tempting to consider artificial means of feeling the high again: drugs, alcohol, shopping, gambling, sex, anorexia, etc. There are many, many options available; most of them wildly unhealthy. It would be dishonest of me to write this particular chronicle without admitting that I have considered maintaining the intoxication through some of these unhealthy, artificial means. Without the crowds and the cheers, the very same emptiness that, in part, fueled my obesity still exists. The surgery did not take that away.

Fortunately (or unfortunately), I have too much knowledge to allow myself to get away with the unhealthiest of stuff for long periods of time. So I move to the healthy side of creating a high. I have tried adventurous, natural-high type activities such as whitewater rafting, kayaking, rollercoasting, snorkeling, and horseback riding. However, the highs of such adventures are short-lived. I don't have the resources nor the time to become a professional daredevil. That's what it would take to keep me excited and focused without becoming bored with the everyday.

The everyday. The crux of it is all is this: I don't deal with normal very well and become bored and restless very easily. I suit up each day, put on my best game face, and go to the stadium. I show up only to find myself playing alone. Occasionally, a few people play along with me, and every now and then there are two or three spectators in the stands. I find myself wanting to go round everyone up again. 'HEY, EVERYONE, c'mon. There's a big game today. Remember? The BIG game. It's still on. It happens every day. It will be fun . . . really . . . umm . . . tickets are free . . . hellooo . . . anybody?' I'm left to figure this out. I have to maintain my weight loss and deal with an emptiness that craves to be filled with either food or excitement. So I'm clueless as to how to do normal, boring, and mundane. It seems completely foreign to me to live the everyday with an occasional spark of spectacular, rather than the spectacular with an occasional spark of normal. Is it possible that part of the solution is to begin to live my life outside of the stadium?

What? Leave the stadium? But I just won the big game!

Yes. Leave I must. And leave I will. The new journey into normal begins. I'm not used to normal. How in the world can that be?

The truth is that the task of being normal isn't over for me. I have to play in that same championship game every single day of my life in order to maintain my weight loss."

This chronicle is phenomenal! The author says it all! She says so many things that many post-ops experience but may be unaware of, unable to put into words, or end up acting out in unhealthy ways. Using her words, let me summarize the incredible message she shares. (Yes, I know you just read her story, but it's so powerful I want you to read a few sentences from it again.)

"It wasn't supposed to be like this. I'm not sure what exactly it was supposed to be like, but this isn't it. How is it that a person can do what seems to be a monumental task, only to find oneself standing in silence? To all concerned, I have reached maintenance weight. However, my disease of chronic morbid obesity is not cured. The disease is merely in remission. It doesn't go away just because my weight 'looks' normal. The surgical tool helps with the battle tremendously and even makes it winnable. But it will never cure the obesity.

There's a huge buildup to weight loss surgery; it is all new, it is all exciting. There were immediate rewards. There was an instant sense of gratification. I've had my fix for the day. I was not prepared for what would happen when the stadium lights went dim and the crowds grew silent. Somehow I had unconsciously come to believe that being thinner would always be fun. It's not. It's just normal. The high that I have been living on is gone. And I still have a battle to fight. This means that one of the toughest parts of normal is that I have to battle my rival without an artificially elevated level of performance-enhancing neurotransmitters. Somehow the foe has to be held at bay for intrinsic reasons.

I'm not sure how to make the transition from stadiums full of cheering fans to a still, small voice inside of myself as the motivation to continue my daily, boring, mundane attempt to hold the line against a rival that will push back at the first opportunity. It is tempting to consider artificial means of feeling the high again: Drugs, alcohol, shopping, gambling, sex, anorexia, etc. Without the crowds and the cheers, the very same emptiness that, in part, fueled my obesity still exists. The surgery did not take that away. The everyday. I'm left to figure this out. I have to maintain my weight loss and deal with an emptiness that craves to be filled with either food or excitement. So I'm clueless as to how to do normal, boring, and mundane.

It seems completely foreign to me to live the everyday with an occasional spark of spectacular, rather than the spectacular with an occasional spark of normal. Is it possible that part of the solution is to begin to live my life outside of the stadium? What? Leave the stadium? But I just won the big game! Yes . . . leave I must. And leave I will. The new journey into normal begins. I'm not used to normal. The truth is that the task of being normal isn't over for me. I have to play in that same championship game every single day of my life in order to maintain my weight loss."

This woman brilliantly highlights the excitement of the weight loss surgery experience. She accurately uses the word "intoxicating" to describe the feelings produced by the excited reactions people have as the weight melts off and a new body emerges. She intuitively knows that she must deal with an emptiness within herself; an emptiness she tried to fill with food and the emptiness that the cheering crowds helped to fill during the weight loss process. She knows, too, that the formerly obese person, whose body changes rapidly after weight loss surgery, is faced with needing to find internal motivation to maintain that healthy new weight. Surgery gets the weight off, but you need to work every day after surgery to keep that weight off. Eating healthy foods, maintaining healthy portions, and daily exercise are required to do that. When the immediate rewards of continual weight loss fade away, and as the cheering of the crowd fades away, you are left with everyday life. No more fuss over your weight loss. Normal life.

Below, a couple of popular WLS bloggers talk about living a "normal" life and being "happy" (or not) after weight loss surgery:

It has nothing to do with food, but it's all about the food.

At some point in our Bariatric After Life™, we learn that our goal is to stop being defined by our surgery and start living life. And yet, we can never forget that we had surgery, because we don't want to return to our old habits. I'll admit, this concept has really tripped me up, because I spend my days reading, writing and talking about bariatrics!

How on earth do I stop thinking about food, when all I think about is food? Throw in a food addiction and, by all rights, I should have a barrel of monkeys on my hands. Only . . . I don't.

How can that be?

Well, in the past few months, I've had the strangest feeling wash over me. It's something akin to "normalcy"—or, as normal as a surgically-altered person can be—and then, not quite normal at all. If I had to define it for you, I believe I would call it: PEACE. Yes, that is it. I am at PEACE within my body. The warring factions have laid down their weapons of mass disruption, and I am now living life on life's terms. Not to confuse PEACE with PERFECTION, or CALMNESS—because neither of those things comes even remotely close.

To be clear, what I am feeling is a reunification or reassociation with mySELF. I have been torn apart for so long, I'd forgotten what it was like to actually BE ME—if I ever really knew at all.

Thanks to therapy and the support of good friends, I now know what it's like (at least as far as anyone can determine) to be ME: It's crazy, fast-paced, gung-ho, exciting, outrageous, magical, frustrating, disconcerting, energizing, exhausting, invigorating, maddening, brilliant, radical, awesome, mellow, unlimited, liberating, compassionate, honest and everything in between. It's like a zoo and a circus and a day at Disneyland, all rolled into one.

For the first time in—probably EVER—I am at home in my own skin, and I like the way it feels. I know what makes me happy, and I know what frustrates me. I know what triggers a binge, and I know what recovery feels like. I know what being fit does for my emotions, and I know what being sick does to my heart. I am in touch with myself and . . . I like me.

Guess what? I am not really about food at all. At least not today. Or yesterday. Maybe I will be tomorrow, I don't know. One thing I do know is, I am hard-pressed to find someone who is not struggling to maintain (or lose) their weight (whether they've had surgery or not); I am hard-pressed to find someone who does not think they *could* workout at least one more day a week (whether they have had surgery or not), and I am hard-pressed to find a person who doesn't wish they hadn't eaten a certain food today (whether they have had surgery or not). So, you see . . . I'm really NOT that different from anybody else, and yet . . . I am.

How? I surround myself by like-minded, successful post-ops.

I get filled up daily by reading inspirational blogs, hearing from my Facebook and Twitter friends, and just chatting it up with healthy, balanced folks. I remain a staunch advocate for spreading the word about the disease of obesity, and I speak to whoever will listen.

If you were to take away one thing from this message, it would be this: The further away from my surgery, the more normal I feel. It's like swimming away from the shore. I can't touch the bottom with my toes anymore, but I'm not freaking out; I'm actually wondering what's beyond that next wave. I never thought that could happen.

Have you ever experienced this?

—Cari De La Cruz (www.bariatricafterlife.com)

You've Lost the Weight.
Why Aren't You Happy?

"I look at the person I photographed in Cabo San Lucas standing on the beach watching the sunset. Is the lady standing out there on the beach happy? Maybe . . . or maybe not. Some might question, 'How could she not be happy standing on the beach and looking at that beautiful sunrise?' Well, the truth is that some people would be standing out there complaining about the sand in their shoes.

Some might also question someone who's been successful with weight loss following surgery, 'How could you not be happy after losing 100, 200, 300, or more pounds?' For people that haven't experienced this, they couldn't possibly understand why some of us aren't happy after surgery and after losing so much weight.

I have stared into the anxious faces of pre-surgical women that long for the simple things like being able to tie their shoes, play with their children, fit in an airplane seat without an extender, and many of the things others take for granted.

We buy into a dream. You know the one . . . where our life becomes this perfect pink cloud of living as a thin person . . . sheer normalcy. No more struggles or pain, everything is rainbows and fairy dust because we lost the weight.

Lately there have been an overwhelming number of posts from unhappy post-ops. If you are one who can relate to this situation, have you asked yourself why you're unhappy? So many people set themselves up for failure because they are SURE that losing the weight will make them instantly happy. I've talked to many pre-ops as they nod their heads and say, 'I understand; all I want is to do normal things.' How can we blame them for wanting more? The first year is made of all these incredible highs from losing weight like we've never lost before! Friends and relatives are telling us how GREAT we look. We get so excited that we can't help but want more! The honeymoon period ends and, unless we are prepared, we may wonder, 'What on earth will I do now to replace those 'bouncing off the wall highs' we have lived for a year?'

We needed to address why we self-medicated with food before we got to this phase—but we certainly have to NOW. Why do you think that having a thin body would make you happy? Think about a friend who has been thin all their lives. I'm pretty sure they don't get out of bed in the morning thinking, 'OH WOW, I'M SO HAPPY BECAUSE I'M THIN!' They are just like everyone else trying to live their life the best they can with the best attitude they can."

Have You Really Forgotten Where You Came From?

Perhaps one of the most useful rituals I do each morning is a walking meditation with my dog. "I am truly grateful for my thin healthy body" (That's the first one followed by many more.) As I'm saying that, I see myself the night before surgery. I remember exactly where I was and I remember to be grateful for where I am today. Is post-op life hard? It is if you believe it is. Wasn't it hard to live in your pre-surgery body? Some of us just can't help ourselves from looking over that fence thinking the grass is greener. I have been discussing this lately but if you really, REALLY think about it, why do you believe that what you want is always in a place you cannot have it? What is the point in that? I will say this again: you have to decide the grass is green enough for right now and when you do, you totally forget you wanted to climb that fence. Even if you do, there's just another fence waiting on the other side. Do you want to enjoy where you are or spend your life climbing fences?

I have found that when I start to see the green grass all around me that the fences fall down because they don't matter any more. After spending 30 years of wanting to be "not obese," I am done with concentrating on what I don't have and am ready to enjoy what I do have! The magic that happens is that you open yourself to the new stuff that can come into your life because your energy is no longer tied up on useless endeavors.

Open your life to new experiences. Quit spending your time concentrating on what you don't have and remember how far you've come. I promise it will make a difference! Try it—you'll like it, Mikey!

Love and Light, Yvonne.

—Yvonne McCarthy (www.wlssuccess.com)

Before weight loss, many obese people report being "obsessed" with food, focusing on diets, endlessly watching the Food Network, obtaining recipes by the hundreds, and talking with family and friends about their weight on a continual basis. This is referred to categorically, as "food porn." It's what helps maintain the focus on food day in and day out. Being food-focused translates to not focusing on real life, real issues, or plain old reality. The contributor readily notes the many vices that can take the place of eating and of food porn that provide a diversion from reality and often provide a temporary high. A high that serves the same purpose that food does: a high that keeps one distracted from reality (the reality of the present—or many times, of the past). Yes—that same past that we think we've moved past, outgrown, or dealt with!

As I have (hopefully) already drilled into your heads, the business of *"learning to live without the cheerleading, without unnatural forms of 'highs'"* is attained by dealing with the past and learning to live in the present. I'm not suggesting that by dealing with the past, you stop focusing on your present. Far from it! You must deal with your present each and every moment! What I'm saying is that in addition to working through any undealt-with issues from your past in therapy, you need to be tending to the present in healthy ways in order to maintain your weight loss.

Dealing with the past and making healthy choices in your present lead to a healthy today and tomorrow.

As a tool for dealing with each and every today, we have the *"Gotta Do 'Ems"*! My list of *"Gotta Do 'Ems"* has been presented to you in a number of ways. Many bariatric programs give patients small cards to carry in their wallets with tips for healthy eating on a daily basis or the "commandments" for maintaining a healthy weight loss. I wrote up the *"Gotta Do 'Ems"* by reading many such lists and compiling those that seemed to be the most consistent in each of the different writings I found. The *"Gotta Do 'Ems"* are sort of the "best of the best" list. I introduced them in my book, *Eat It Up!* and they are as follows:

MAKE CONSISTENTLY HEALTHY FOOD CHOICES
Protein first plus a vegetable or fruit

MAINTAIN PORTION CONTROL
Forevermore in every eating situation

EXERCISE ON A REGULAR BASIS
That means *daily*

DRINK PLENTY OF WATER THROUGHOUT THE DAY
But *not* 30 minutes before or after meals

EAT BREAKFAST
Protein, protein, protein . . .
doesn't have to be traditional breakfast food

PLAN YOUR MEALS AND FOLLOW YOUR PLAN
You don't have to want to . . . you just have to!

KEEP A FOOD DIARY
It keeps you accountable
and is the best way to maintain weight loss.

KEEP AN EXERCISE DIARY
It will remind you of all the great hard work you are doing.

GET ENOUGH SLEEP
Who knew there was a connection between sleep and weight? There is!

UTILIZE A HEALTHY SUPPORT SYSTEM
Participate in local and online support groups.

PARTICIPATE IN INDIVIDUAL AND/OR GROUP THERAPY
Okay . . . not a daily thing,
but a very good idea on a weekly basis.

(To obtain free copies of the *"Gotta Do 'Ems,"* print them from my website at www.conniestapletonphd.com. You can use the list as a daily check-off or simply as a way to keep the essential behavioral tasks in mind by posting them on your fridge and other places where you will see them frequently.)

The *"Gotta Do 'Ems"* are the behavioral components of maintaining your weight loss. One of the contributors in this book noted, *"For me, bariatric surgery is like a three-legged stool. The top of the stool is bariatric surgery; the three legs consist of eating habits, exercise, and support."* I often use the analogy of weight loss surgery being a three-legged stool as well. I combine her eating habits and exercise into a "Behavioral" component as one of the legs. For me, the other two are "Therapy (addressing underlying issues and obtaining support)" and "Changin' Stinkin' Thinkin'."

The "Changin' Stinkin' Thinkin'" leg of the stool is critical, as are implementing behavior changes (the *"Gotta Do 'Ems"*) and the therapy legs. (One additional note about the therapy part: included in the therapy section is the need for support, which many of the contributors to this book have noted. The Post-Op

& the Doc (www.apostopandadoc.com) say this about weight loss: "No one can do it for you. But you can't do it alone." It takes a lot of support to maintain the behaviors necessary to keep your weight off. Support comes in the form of the people at your bariatric center, support group meetings, online WLS friends, therapists, and *genuinely supportive* family and friends.

Now, back to the Stinkin' Thinkin,' which is just what it sounds like. Thinking that stinks! Thoughts like, "Why bother with this healthy eating?" "I blew it already today. I'll start over on. . . ." "I'm too tired/busy/bored/sad/happy/stressed, etc., etc., to exercise." This sort of thinking stinks! It leads to feeling badly and then to poor behaviors that result in extra pounds.

An entire book could be dedicated to the importance of changin' stinkin' thinkin' to positive thinking (in fact, several books have been written on that topic!). The following paragraphs are from my first book, *Eat It Up!*

> Thoughts lead to feelings and to behavior. You will need to learn to recognize what you do with your thoughts. If the thoughts are negative, you can dwell on them if you want to feel badly. You can opt to find a more positive way to frame the thoughts, thereby feeling better. Your behavior will follow suit, depending on whether you focus on negative or positive thoughts.
>
> As the Swedish proverb says, "Those who wish to sing, always find a song". Think about the things you have said to yourself lately. I'm betting there have been comments like, "You idiot!" "Why did I eat all of that?" "God, I'm so stupid. How could I have done that?" "I'm such a loser" "What was I thinking?" "I'm ugly." "I'm fat." Most of us don't run around sharing those thoughts out loud, but we often have an ongoing narrative of negative comments about ourselves streaming through our brains. Our negative self-talk can be like a train that has no caboose; it never seems to end.
>
> Here's a challenge I pose to clients and am now presenting to you. I ask you: "Would you say the negative statements above to your very best friend?" Think about it. Your lifelong soul-sister calls you up, four months after having bariatric surgery,

and says to you, "I can't believe what I did today. A co-worker brought in my favorite chocolate fudge cake and throughout the day I managed to eat three pieces of it. I feel horrible—physically and emotionally." Is this what you would say to her: "Wow! You're really a loser! How stupid can you be? I can't believe you let yourself eat three pieces of chocolate cake after what you have been through! What were you thinking?"

Come on now. You would never in a million years do that to your best friend! More likely you would say something along the lines of: "I can hear how upset you are with yourself. I know you are feeling horrible right now. Let's talk about it. You have been really diligent about what you have been eating since you had surgery. Your health is important to you. Eating that cake obviously wasn't in your best interest. It's not like you have regularly overindulged like that since having your surgery. There must be something going on. What was bothering you?" You would kindly talk to your friend about the circumstances surrounding her eating too much cake. You would help her remain accountable for her behavior, but you would not beat her up for it.

The challenge to you is to treat yourself as kindly as you would your best friend. This includes talking to yourself as gently as you would your best friend, even when you need to hold yourself accountable. In other words, when friends come to us, they are looking for affirmation and validation of their feelings. Good friends want to be supported and encouraged by the people they love and trust. They also want to be gently held accountable for their behavior. The second response above is one that demonstrates good listening and good friendship skills. You can practice these same skills of good listening and good friendship with yourself as well as with those you love.

Positive Behaviors + Therapy/Support + Positive Thinking = Sustained Weight Loss

This chapter is about living the Bariatric After Life and the things you "gotta do" to maintain a healthy weight. The equation above is one you might consider tattooing along your forearm! Okay—just print it out from your computer and post it around your house. This is the formula for sustained weight loss success!

This insightful, humorous contributor speaks of how she works
this formula in her everyday life:

"I came into this world weighing 11 pounds, 6 ounces, and
only lost weight when I had a bowel movement. At least that's
my father's story. Unfortunately, not much changed for my
entire adolescent and young adult life, because I continued to
lose weight the same way. For the record, my mom developed
gestational diabetes with me, gained about 100 pounds, and was
three weeks overdue. Trust me, they do NOT allow such a long
period of time to pass before delivering babies anymore.

When I look at my first baby picture from the hospital (not the
one of the ugly little boy that they mistakenly gave my mom), I
am mortified. Staring back from the faded black and white photo
is a chubby, cross-eyed little girl with fluffy cheeks and a very
confused look on her face. I think I remained that way for about
40 years.

My mother reports that I had the umbilical cord wrapped
around my neck three times (which could explain my bloated
head), but my father said I arrived rear-end first, and you really
can't blame THAT fluffiness on the umbilical cord. It's true—they
did call me 'Rump and Silk Skin' for as long as I can remember,
and my substantial derriere seemed to have a life of its own,
especially in grade school. I was the little girl with the bonus butt.
They even wrote a poem about me:

> Roses are red.
> Violets are blue.
> Her butt is as big
> As a B-52.

Clever, huh? The worst part was, I couldn't tell my parents
because we did NOT use the word 'butt' in our house. It was
always referred to as the hindquarters, derriere, rear end or but-
tocks. Forest Gump would have been right at home with my
mom and her box of chocolates.

I grew up looking at life through 'Shasta-bottom glasses'
(because we didn't drink sugar Coke). I always thought I was fat,
though in retrospect, I can clearly see that I wasn't. When you
believe something as strongly as I did, you can see how easy it

was for everyone ELSE to believe it, too. I was fat and homely, and if word got out that I had a crush on a boy, he became the laughingstock of his group. Why? Because he was the guy who was adored by the girl with the bubble butt.

I was taller than the other girls and had a much different shape. I always had curves where they had 'straightaways,' and I started wearing a bra in sixth grade. I remember one incident from fifth grade, where the teacher thought it would be a brilliant idea to have us all MEASURE and WEIGH ourselves. Why this seemed like the perfect educational opportunity is beyond me, but I gamely participated (because, in those days, you weren't allowed to be a conscientious objector.)

I think I was about 5'2" or 5'3", but none of that mattered, because I weighed 108 pounds. That was about 30 pounds more than just about everybody else. My head circumference was also spectacularly grand, measuring 14.75" around. There were other body parts measured, but the only two numbers I remember are the distance around my skull and the weight of me, my big butt, and my thunderous thighs. Naturally, everyone in the class saw my humiliation and did what all compassionate humans do: they broadcast it to the rest of the school. I wasn't smart enough to tell them that my head measurement was directly correlative to the size of my brain (and thus, my intelligence), nor did I share with them that I would SIT ON THEM if they didn't shut up. No. I just sat back and ate up the ridicule. Along with a 13-cent candy bar and an 8-cent ice cream sundae from the corner drugstore. Every day.

But, don't get me wrong. My family was incredibly supportive, especially my big (type 1 diabetic) brother who was a beanpole, by virtue of his disease. The 'benefit' was that he couldn't gain weight—even if he wanted to. The worst part was, he acted like he had something to do with it. Of course, now I know that this was probably a show of bravado for having to live with such a horrible burden, but in those days, I would actually dream of 'contracting' the same thing, just so I could be skinny, too. How embarrassing.

Meanwhile, my dad would just tell me to 'ignore' anyone who made fun of me, my mom would sew many of my clothes (because she knew just how to alter things to fit), my grandma would tell me to 'slow down' or 'stop eating between meals,' and my grandpa would remark about the size of my generous 'shirt pockets.'

Yes, home is where the heart is, and I swear, if I'd been any more loved, I'd have weighed 400 pounds, rather than 300-plus, by the time I had my bariatric surgery.

I can't really blame my mother, though, because she fed us incredibly healthy foods, didn't allow snacking, always packed our lunches, and did NOT stock the pantry with junk food of any sort.

I hated her for that.

The only time we got anything remotely resembling the junk food that my friends ate was the very first week of the school year, when we would enjoy Hunt's chocolate pudding cups and Fritos in our lunch boxes. When we went camping each summer, we also got JUNK cereal (instead of Spoon Size Shredded Wheat). You know those variety packs in the little boxes? Oddly, I never got the Fruit Loops, Cap'n Crunch, Cocoa Puffs, Lucky Charms, or Trix. No. I got the Cheerios, Rice Krispies, and Raisin Bran. For someone who couldn't eat sugar because of his diabetes, my brother ate a lot of sugar, and my mother turned a blind eye.

I've discussed this in therapy and finally made the connection when I was mentioning my propensity for bingeing on Fruit Loops. Clearly, I am compensating for all of those camping trips.

Anyway, aside from the few indiscretions, my mom always ensured that our plates were filled with healthy foods in proper portions. My dad always ensured that I ate all of that healthy food in proper portions—even if it meant I stayed at the table, staring mournfully at the bunch of broccoli, pile of Brussels sprouts, puddle of peas, or bowl of pickled beets. Sometimes, my dad would 'take pity' on me, and allow me to leave the table with the veggies unfinished. Odd how I never had trouble finishing my potatoes, rice, or elbow macaroni.

We did not eat dessert—except on special occasions—and somewhere along the way, I must have determined that, like Scarlett O'Hara, I would 'never go hungry again'—at least not where sugary foods and white starchy carbs were concerned. No one would ever steal my Fruit Loops and I would NEVER be forced to eat broccoli again. Needless to say, food was confusing in my house. Yummy food (like cake or cookies) was something to fear and hide, while healthy food was something to despise and suffer through.

Did I mention that my mother was one of the very first Weight Watchers in our area? Yes. She made it to goal and received a diamond-encrusted 'W' pin that made her a lifetime member and entitled her to free meetings forever. I loved that pin, but she didn't wear it very much. Probably because she didn't keep the weight off, though she was a serial Weight Watchers group lurker.

You see, just because my mom fed US healthy food, didn't mean SHE was a healthy eater. Au contraire; there was always a container of rocky road ice cream in the freezer (which I left alone because I didn't like walnuts). She was always dispatching my dad to buy her chocolate (something I never completely understood). All I knew was, before the chocolate, she was mean, and after the chocolate, she was . . . fat. At least that's how she always saw herself. I thought she was beautiful (and so did all of my friends and all of my dad's co-workers). She had the most stunning red hair and always dressed modestly. My father adored her until the day he died, and I loved her frosty peach lipstick. I would spend hours watching her expertly apply her make-up, color her hair, or style it like Carol Brady, and never missed an opportunity to vehemently announce that I would never color my hair OR wear make-up because I was a natural beauty—just like her. My mom was a classy and talented lady, who never believed it.

But, enough about mom; back to me.

I grew up in a time when kids were meant to go outside and play, so I was extremely active. I rode my bike everywhere (because it was my 'car'), and if I wasn't riding it, I was skating to the mall (or doing a 'skate-by' of a very cute boy's house). I was on the softball team, I loved kickball, but hated dodge ball (because I was a very easy target). My mother was always shooing me outside to play touch football with the neighborhood kids, draw chalk hopscotches on the sidewalk, or do gymnastics (like Nadia Comaneci) on the neighbor's grass. I also loved to play hide-and-go-seek, or go for strolls around the block, singing Beatles songs at the top of my lungs. So, you see, I didn't sit still very often.

So, why was I fat? Though we have now established that I really wasn't 'fat,' I WAS in the 'overweight' category on the doctor's weight graph, I did have trouble finding pants that fit, and I could never pass the Presidential Physical Fitness tests in PE. To this day, I fear sit-ups, have never done a chin-up, and am firmly convinced that I could not run away from a turtle. All of these realities combined—nay—conspired to fill my head with visions of fatness.

Oh, I know my mom said that I wasn't fat—merely zaftig, voluptuous, and substantial, but none of my friends fit those adjectives, and besides, there was never a big enough bathing suit at anyone's house, so I couldn't spontaneously jump into the pool with everyone else. Speaking of, I only made it to Tadpole 3 in swim class (and I flunked that twice.) The instructor said I was a 'nice girl,' but 'couldn't swim her way out of a puddle.' I had to face facts: I was a floater, not a sinker, and I couldn't swim. What I did was euphemistically referred to as 'controlled drowning.'

And all of it took place wearing the most humiliating bathing suits you've ever seen. Of course, I couldn't fit junior suits and had to wear old-lady ones, and I wouldn't be caught DEAD at the beach. When I wore shorts, they would ride up in the middle and if I wasn't 'picking them' out of my rear, I was tugging them down over my thighs. I never understood why my friends' shorts didn't do the same thing, until I lost enough weight to experience the 'thrill' of thighs that didn't meet in the middle and create enough friction to start any discriminating Boy Scout's fire. Suffice it to say, summer was NOT my favorite season.

Now, I don't want you to think that I was antisocial, because I did have friends. Little friends; the kind who were nowhere near my size. I was an Amazon who always ended up at the bottom of the 'people pyramid.' We could never share clothes—unless they needed a 'sleep shirt,' which I could always provide.

Remember when Levi's 501's were all the rage? Remember how that leather tag on the back clearly showed your size? Yes, I realize they were made for boys (who don't have hips), but how could I explain that my waist was smaller than my friend's 28, when I had to hide it in size 33's (with the waist taken way in, thank you, Mom).

I learned pretty quickly to be the funny, creative girl that everybody could like. I drew cartoons for the popular kids and told jokes to the unpopular ones (my friends). I was insanely jealous of the girls who wore Chemin de fer, Jordache, or Ditto jeans, and nothing came between me and my Calvins—mostly, because Calvins didn't fit, but also because they were too expensive for my parents to buy. In a sense, it was fortunate for them that I was fat. And, let's not talk about my PE uniform. The one with the bloomers that didn't. They did not make knee socks long enough to cover my embarrassing thighs, and my mother was forever making comments about how ridiculous I looked with my 'socks pulled up so high.'

I was terrified to go to parties because I was just sure everyone was talking about me (and my big butt, and my long socks). Orthodontia only magnified the problem, and a bottom retainer did amazing things for my lisp. Great. In a sense, I finally resembled one of the Bradys—Cindy, not Carol.

And then I shed that baby fat. Just in time, I might add, to enter high school. My sophomore year was incredible. I got down to 143 pounds (by getting sick), but I had the cutest wardrobe ever. I had enviable hair, wore fashionable clothes, and was a trend-setter. My biggest problem was how to keep the angora hair off my corduroy pants. I danced to the Go-Go's, the B-52's and the Stray Cats. I had my first boyfriend (and my first kiss). I was pretty and popular (in the third tier, anyway—just below the cheerleaders and the 'easy girls'), but I was still fat and I still couldn't run a mile as fast as everyone else . . . or bunny-hop the bleacher stairs . . . or survive the leg-lift for a whole minute.

I was a failure AND I was fat.

My saving grace was my brains. I had always been smart, but now I was in advanced placement courses, so I was among the upper echelon of smart people. I had to work just to keep up with them. Thus began my inferiority-superiority complex— a little game I liked to play, where I made sure the slightly less smart people knew how brilliant I was and the brilliant people knew how little I cared. I gained back 10 pounds that year.

So, if I was so smart, and people thought I was pretty, why didn't I believe them?

It has taken me a long time to begin to figure this out, and losing half of my body weight didn't magically make all of my hang-ups go away. It's only in recent years that I have begun to acknowledge and talk about some painful and ugly episodes from my past.

Like so many obese people, I was sexually abused as a child. Once, around age three-and-a-half, by the 'kind' next-door neighbor's brother; once, at age seven, by the neighborhood child who was abused herself, and once, at age 10, by my big brother. I won't get into the gory details, as they are ugly and a little murky. I will simply say that the events served to reinforce the errant belief that I couldn't or shouldn't defend myself, that I probably did something to deserve the abuse, and that I wasn't like every other victim.

You see, I didn't harbor a bunch of pent-up anger—at least not to my knowledge— and I didn't have a problem expressing myself in a healthy, sexual way with my husband. In my estimation, I had survived unscathed.

But nothing could be further from the truth, because I ate the humiliation. I ate the feeling of being out of control. I ate the unbearable disappointment in my brother. I ate and ate and ate to take the pain away, but I only hurt more, and I didn't understand WHY.

Before my surgery, if you'd asked whether I'd come from a dysfunctional family, I'd have quickly and confidently told you, 'no.' If you asked why I moved into my own apartment when I was 18, I'd have firmly told you it was because I was wildly independent. I would not have thought to tell you that I was running away from my crazy mother, who, I am now convinced is bipolar, but was then simply locked in a mental ward and diagnosed with extreme PMS after threatening suicide. You haven't lived until you've watched your father break down the bedroom door to reach your histrionic mother, and you haven't lived until she suffocated you by living every moment of your life with and for you because she was so desperate to have control.

I don't want to sound bitter, and I never believed that I was bitter. After all, my parents were married for 47 years (until my dad's death parted them in 2009); my father was brilliant and worked hard to provide for us; my mother was a stay-at-home mom who always had dinner on the table at 5 o'clock, and was the envy of all of my friends; they were always generous with their love and affection—to me and my brother, and with each other. There were rules to follow and consequences to pay. We were spanked with a wooden spoon for serious infractions, but I never viewed that as abuse, and still don't. It's true that my dad broke a chair over my brother's back, but I believed he deserved it because he was unbelievably disrespectful to my dad and said horrible, angry things to him. Maybe I adopted that opinion as retribution for what he did to me. I don't know. The idea that they did not physically abuse us might be open to debate, but I knew that my parents never 'whipped' me or hit me hard, and I DID learn my lesson.

Or maybe I just learned to eat to cover the pain. I'm not sure.

All I know is, my family, for all of its flaws, was not something I would characterize as the cause of my obesity—unless you want to blame genetics. Well, that has long been my contention, anyway. My parents loved me, but they made mistakes, as all parents do. I don't find particular need to BLAME them for my wounds, but as an adult, I do find that I struggle to have a healthy relationship with both my brother and my mother. Perhaps I am still feeding my guilt and grief, each time I binge? I'm not sure, but that's what therapy is for.

In the final analysis, this is what I have learned:

Many of my behaviors as an adult came from misinterpreted, misunderstood, and mischaracterized incidents when I was child. Of course, when you are 5 or 10, you don't interpret things from an adult perspective. You can't, because you haven't lived enough yet. All you can do is react, usually on a primal, defensive level. All you can do is believe that you are the problem—not the person you love and who you believe loves you; not the person who you believe is smart enough not to make mistakes, and not the person who you refuse to believe could ever be wrong or hurt you. It's is only after a few years of therapy (and about 20 years of messing up—uh, parenting my own child) that I am able to see how loving people can easily ruin people they love.

There is no single cause of obesity, any more than there is a single cure. The best I can hope for is healing of painful childhood memories, and strengthening of my adult future."

I love how this contributor notes that she *was* loved by her parents. They did not intentionally try to harm her in any way. That's true for almost all parents. We (parents) don't (usually) do things knowing they will be hurtful or harmful to our children. It doesn't mean that sometimes kids aren't hurt by things we do or say. What this contributor teaches us is that it is our responsibility to deal with whatever our issues are, regardless of where they stem from. As adults we need to take responsibility for our lives. No matter what happened in our childhood, we are responsible for creating the quality of our adult life. So, whatever you need to do in order to be able to follow through with making healthy choices, asking for help, and learning to think positively, it is up to you to take the steps to do those things!

Asking for help is something many people have trouble doing. The man who shared the next story speaks about the importance of doing just that:

"I achieved my goal of having bariatric surgery in July of 2011. Now, in February of 2012, I've lost over 110 pounds. I'm wearing clothes and clothing sizes I haven't been able to wear in more than 15 years. I am doing things and planning on doing things I haven't done in at least that long, if not longer.

Many people ask me how long it took from the time I first entered the bariatric program until I had my surgery done. They're usually astounded when I tell them it was over nine years. Their first question is usually 'Did you have some health issues that kept you from having the surgery?' Nope. The health issues I did have—hypertension, sleep apnea, and gout, all just made me more of a candidate for the surgery. 'Did you have some problem with your health insurance or finances that made getting this done a problem?' Again, negative. My health insurance covered everything from the operation, to my hospital stay, to all of my meds. So why the hell did it take me so long to get through this and get it done? Well, it's a little thing I like to call 'The Masculine Facade.'

As men, in our culture, we're raised seeing very 'manly' images. We saw John Wayne and Clint Eastwood, the lone gunslingers riding in to clean up a crooked town, relying on nothing and no one but their wits, their brawn, and their trusty six-shooter. We're shown images of Sly Stallone in the original First Blood, sewing up a huge gash in his own arm without making a sound or even having a painful look on his face. Right! Most of us guys whine like babies if we get so much as a paper cut. But I was a typical American male, and as such, usually ignored what I was doing to myself and refused to ask for anyone's help.

I had been at my job for more than two years with full health care benefits before I ever connected with a primary care physician. The only time I ever went to a doctor was if I had a worker's comp issue and went to the ER. I knew I had to get a handle on my weight, but I was a man, after all! I had to go it on my own or I couldn't call myself a real man

Eventually, I broke down and scheduled an appointment with my PCP and asked about a weight loss program. I expected to hear DIET. I expected to hear EXERCISE. I expected to hear CHANGE OF HABITS. I never expected to hear the word SUR-GERY. When I did hear that word—to say that I balked is an understatement. I became like the Mexican bandit in 'The Trea-sure of the Sierra Madre.' Surgery? I didn't need no stinking sur-gery! I was a MAN, damn it! I could handle this by myself. Well, guess what, boys and girls, friends, Romans, and countrymen? I was wrong. And it took a lot of time (years, in fact), love, sup-port, and—as much as it pained me to admit I needed it and then subject myself to it—counseling, to figure that indeed, I could not handle it myself.

In the interest of keeping this short and sweet, I won't tell you all the bloody gory details of my issues. It's enough to let you know that I had issues. I had things going on in my head and yes, in my heart, that had me eating too much of too many unhealthy foods and drinking way too much beer. (I like an occa-sional taste of Jack Daniel's, but I'm primarily a beer guy.) I had to get it through my thick, masculine skull that I needed help to get healthy. But before I could do that I needed to admit three things to myself:

- One, that there was no shame in admitting that I couldn't do this on my own.

- Two, that I did have issues and that I needed help rec-ognizing and dealing with them. And,

- Three, that I wasn't as tough as I thought I was, and that it really was okay for me not to be tough.

I'm more than seven months out from out from surgery now. In these seven months things have changed in ways I could have never anticipated. But some things have stayed the same. I still have days when I have to battle my demons. And ya know what? Some days I lose. But these days, I win a little more often than I used to. And on the days I lose, I learn things about myself, and about those nasty little guys that help me to win the next time around."

My very sincere thanks to this man for presenting another male perspective and for illustrating the importance of recognizing that we all need help. I've said it before and I'll say it again: "Weight loss. No one can do it for you but you can't do it alone."

I work with numerous pre- and post-ops on therapeutic issues in individual sessions. I also require the patients I see for pre-surgical evaluations to watch a video I put together, informing them of some critical information they need prior to having weight loss surgery. (This is also very relevant information after surgery, so if you haven't seen it, you can watch it on my website www.conniesta-pletonphd.com—in three episodes—or on my YouTube channel [www.youtube.com/user/ConnieStapletonPhD]) and watch the eight shorter videos. The material is the same, and I sincerely do encourage you to watch these. Great information and it's all free! In these videos, I note the following points:

> "It is vital that you change the relationship you have with food. You may not even realize what the nature of your relationship with food is until after you have the surgery. When food is no longer available to you in the way it has been before the procedure, you discover more about what your relationship with food is. Therefore, you may need to have this talk again at some point after the surgery. However, we have to start with where you are at the present time.
>
> Here is what you are going to do. Determine a time when no one else is going to be around to disrupt you. Go into the kitchen and open the refrigerator door wide open. Do the same with the freezer. Then open every cupboard that has food in it, and every drawer that holds snacks or goodies. Then, with all the doors wide open so you can see the food, talk to it—out loud—and say something like this:
>
> "Well, food. I'm having this talk with you today for an extremely important reason. Oreos, pay attention. I'm speaking directly to you. Potato chips—you, too. And all of the rest of you. For a long time, you and I have had a very close relationship. You have been my friend. I have turned to you in times of loneliness, happiness, frustration, fear, and boredom.

You know we have done some damage on those long winter afternoons when there wasn't much else to do. Yep—you were there with me, keeping me company during every football game for the last many years. You and I have spent a lot of time together reading sappy romance novels. When I was mad at my spouse (or mother or children or boss) you were always just a few steps away. Yep—we go way back. The time has come, however, for our relationship to change.

"You remember when my best friend, Brenda from work, and I had a falling out last year? You should remember, I ate and ate and ate about it. I ate when I was mad at her. I ate when I was sad about the situation with her. I thought she had been the best friend I had ever had. Then I learned that she was really a back-stabber. She was talking about me behind my back to all of our other friends. I had to make a decision about what to do with the relationship. We work together so I couldn't just cut her out of my life. I decided to let her know that I was hurt by her actions and I have since chosen to limit my interactions with her. Well, it's sort of the same with you and me, food. I counted on you to be there for me at all times. And you have been! But, like Brenda, you have sort of turned on me as a friend.

"Look at me! I'm tremendously overweight. I have pain in my knees due to my weight. My blood pressure and cholesterol are skyrocketing, and I'm on the verge of being diabetic. To my way of thinking then, food, our relationship has become detrimental to me. Therefore, it has to change. I don't foresee you taking charge of the situation, so I am going to have to. I still want and need you in my life. But I want ours to be a healthy relationship. I know that I have abused you. It isn't really that you have done anything intentional to hurt me. But I have let that happen between us. I allowed a perfectly natural relationship become toxic. It's time for that to change. In order for us to have a healthy relationship, I need to think of you in a different way and to interact with you in a different way. From now on, you and I are going to be respectful to one another. I am not going to abuse you by using you to deal with my feelings. I am going to treat you like you were intended to be treated: as a means to keep my body healthy.

"Yep—I am going to eat to live from now on. I have lived to eat for such a long time. I abused you and in return, you have harmed me. Not any more. We are entering a new, healthy relationship. You are going to be a good friend to me and keep my body healthy. I am also going to be a better friend to myself and set limits with you. I'm going to have to learn to set limits with others too, because not doing so may be part of the reason I turned to you in the first place.

"I sometimes let other people take advantage of me and then I would harm myself by eating too much. From now on, food, it's eat to live! So, Oreos, chips, ice cream, mashed potatoes, rice, and candy. We shall meet on an extremely limited basis from here on out. Some of you may never be allowed in this house again. I do thank you for having kept me company for so long, but it is time I say good-bye to some of you. Others of you may visit on occasion, but it will be rare. I appreciate that I had you to turn to at times. In the future, however, I will find more adaptive ways to spend my free time and healthier ways to deal with my emotions.

"In the next several weeks, I may have to talk with you again. I may find myself grieving the loss of you as I did the loss of my friendship with Brenda. I have survived that loss, and I shall survive the loss of you, unhealthy food. In summary, I am redefining my relationship with you as of this moment. You are now my source of fuel and energy for my body. I look forward to our new healthy relationship."

You may feel like a complete fool doing this, but you may also find that doing so establishes a determined mindset from which you operate from that moment on. After your CTR (Changing the Relationship) talk with food, whenever you are temped by cookies or cake or potato chips, you can say (out loud or to yourself), "I'm sorry, but as I told you before, our relationship has changed. Cookies, you are not necessary for my survival, and you do nothing to add to my good health. Therefore, I will choose to leave you alone and will instead choose to have yogurt." Every time you think thoughts like this, you are making a commitment to yourself to choose to be healthy. The consequences of such a choice are feeling better about yourself for doing what's best for you and making a healthy choice for your body.

The CTR talk with food is one of the ways you learn HOW to make healthy choices with food. It is a tool you can use at times when you are tempted to eat the wrong things. Remember, the goal is to KEEP the weight off after you lose it.

I obtained permission from two people I work with in therapy to share some brief examples of work they are doing as they prepare for weight loss surgery! Hear me again—these are both *pre-ops* who understand the importance of addressing their lifelong issues, either directly or indirectly related to food, in order to make the process of making healthy behavioral choices easier after their surgeries.

The first thing I'll share is something I encourage everyone to do: Write a letter to food. Everybody has some sort of relationship with food. For some people, the relationship they have with food is closer and more emotionally intimate than the relationships they have with most people. For some, the relationship is strictly a business exchange: "I eat you, and you keep my body moving." It's important to figure out what role food plays in your life. This information will help you recognize how easy or difficult the change in your relationship with food will be following surgery. The more emotionally connected you are to food, the more you depend on food. The more you cherish that relationship, the more difficult it will be to change that relationship to one of a healthy, mutually respectful relationship after surgery. In a healthy relationship with food, you say to food, "I need you to keep my body healthy and strong, which is why I eat you." Food, in return says, "Okay. I can do that if you agree to choose carefully from my many options. If you do your part by choosing healthy options (protein first; lots of fruits and vegetables; steamed, grilled, and broiled foods; and 'real, unprocessed' foods, then I will do my part in helping make you healthy and strong."

Read the following letter from a patient to food. Pay attention to how you feel while you are reading it. Note what emotions are stirred in you.

> Dear Food,
>
> At times you've seemed like my friend. You've comforted me and brought me joy. You and I have spent a lot of time together. However, I think I love you much more than you love me.
>
> I actually obsess about you. I think about you all the time. You, on the other hand, while you do comfort me and bring me joy, also provide me with unwanted pounds, cholesterol, high blood sugar, and overall bad health. So what's a girl to do?
>
> I need to find something to replace you. It will be hard... I'm sure. Nonetheless, it must be done. I doubt that you will care at all. After all, you are pretty fickle. You'll take up with anyone who has an appetite or suffers from "down in the dumps blues."
>
> I'm sure that they'll love you, as did I. Well, maybe not as much as me, but you'll put them under your spell before long. They'll think that you're a wonderful part of their life. This will continue for years—until it's too late. The pounds will be there and will remain very difficult to shed. It's so hard to say good-bye to someone that has been such a huge part of my life for over fifty years.
>
> I wish we could just go to divorce court. I would let you have all of the assets; I wouldn't put up a fight. The pounds could be given to someone else without regret from me.
>
> I'm sure that I will miss you. It is going to be hard; more difficult than anything I've ever done in my life. However, as the song says, 'I will survive.' My life without you WILL be fulfilling. I have to make it that way with other "friends" and "lovers." So, good-bye food. Please leave without a fuss. I won't change my mind.
>
> Your Former Lover and Best Friend,
> Patient

Let me substitute just a few words from her letter. Read it and again, note how you feel as you do.

> Dear Abusive Boyfriend/Husband,
>
> At times you've seemed like my friend. You've comforted me and brought me joy. You and I have spent a lot of time together. However, I think I love you much more than you love me.

I actually obsess about you. I think about you all the time. You, on the other hand, while you do comfort me and bring me joy, also provide me with unwanted tears, anger, frustration and doubt—about us and about myself. So what's a girl to do?

I need to find someone healthy to replace you. It will be hard, I'm sure. Nonetheless, it must be done. I doubt that you will care at all. After all, you are pretty fickle. You'll take up with anyone who has an appetite or suffers from "down in the dumps blues."

I'm sure that they'll love you, as did I. Well, maybe not as much as me, but you'll put them under your spell before long. They'll think that you're a wonderful part of their life. This will continue for years—until it's too late. It's so hard to say good-bye to someone that has been such a huge part of my life for over fifty years.

I wish we could just go to divorce court. I would let you have all of the assets; I wouldn't put up a fight. The pain could be given to someone else without regret from me.

I'm sure that I will miss you. It is going to be hard; more difficult than anything I've ever done in my life. However, as the song says, 'I will survive.' My life without you WILL be fulfilling. I have to make it that way with other "friends" and "lovers." So, good-bye, Tom (Brad, George, Matt). Please leave without a fuss. I won't change my mind.

Your Former Lover and Best Friend,
Patient

Do you get it? I changed approximately a dozen words. The letter *she wrote to food* is ridiculously similar to a letter that one could write to a partner in an unhealthy relationship! We all know stories of people who stay in unhealthy relationships for a long time—usually, way too long. The "victim" of the story, whether male or female, will claim they stay in the unhealthy relationship because they "love" the abuser. (Trust me, that is *not* love.) The truth is, they are *dependent upon* this person. And many people are *dependent upon* food to "make them feel better." Not everyone's letter to food would sound like a love letter, but everyone who has issues with food has some emotional relationship with food. Write your letter to food. See what you can learn about yourself and your relationship with food. If you need to, take it with you and go see a professional therapist. Or talk to a good friend about it. You're certain to learn some interesting things about your relationship with food.

In another letter to food, a patient writes in a practical manner, with a take-charge attitude:

> Dear Food,
> I really don't know how to say goodbye to you. Truth is, I haven't got a clue. I need you to live, but I also need you less to really live fully, as you are killing me. I really love you and have depended on you for comfort as long as I can remember. I have, however, used you for comfort and for all the wrong reasons! I know it's time for me to let go of you, and the hold you have over me and my life! I can't live my life anymore based on what the next meal is going to be or which sweet treat I get to eat next! I have to start using you for nourishment and health reasons instead of using you as my own personal drug of choice. The worst thing about you is that I literally need you to live—so I can't give you up completely. But I can learn how to set limits with you and impose boundaries so that we can learn to be friends instead of enemies! Because, frankly, you are my best friend and worst enemy! I hate the way our relationship has been, and I want to change it. I need to make it better so that we can live out the rest of our lives together in harmony! It's going to be rough, and I'm not sure how to go about this yet, but I'm learning, and I'm ready to finally say goodbye! Thanks for being there, but thanks even more for leaving!
> Sincerely,
> Me

Write letters to food every couple of months. Take note of how that relationship is changing over time. Hopefully, food becomes a means of providing your body with the nourishment it needs to help you get through your life in as good of shape as possible. You've heard the analogy about your body being like a car. If you spent a hundred thousand dollars on a car, you would hopefully put the best grade gas in the tank to keep the car running as efficiently and as smoothly as possible. Remember—you are a top of the line model and as such, your engine deserves the best possible fuel (the healthy stuff)!

The next series of entries is written by a male patient *prior* to his weight loss surgery. Please keep that in mind as you read his food entries. These would not be in line with what a post-op eats. I chose to keep the food selections in so you could reflect back and see that you may have eaten similarly. Although this man is preparing for weight loss surgery and believes he is making healthy food choices, the foods he chooses are sometimes quite unhealthy (hot dogs, fries). The important points in reading these entries are to 1) note his positive attitude, 2) note his willingness to admit when he is not feeling positive, 3) note how he makes a commitment to move forward if he's doing something less than optimal toward his goals, and 4) note his clearly stated, measurable exercise goals.

Daily Log

January 24, 2012

Starting this daily log of my activities and food intake should have been done weeks ago. That being said, I am starting the log now because I feel it is time for me to do so. I have seen my therapist three times, and I feel it has really done me some good. Since our last session I have had good days and bad days. It was during this time I made a realization and learned something. Some people say that setbacks are inevitable; however, you rarely hear how hard it is to bounce back from these setbacks. This is something I have learned firsthand since my last session. I became upset and depressed because of issues involving my dad and brother and did a bad thing by stopping at Burger King. The following few days were more difficult to do the right thing. I am glad that I have been able to suppress the bad habit again. What did I learn? When someone has an addiction it is an everyday battle. I must always be vigilant and strong in my pursuit of making a better life. To be honest, until someone experiences it firsthand, most people will not or cannot understand how difficult fighting an addiction is.

While I do admit that the setback I had is bad, I prefer to look at it like this, "If I had not had a setback now, I would not understand how difficult it is to recover from it." Today I am feeling much better and have started getting into a real rhythm.

My meals for today include lunch: two peanut butter and jelly sandwiches with one serving of fries. Dinner was one chicken breast with green beans and for dessert, sugar-free Jell-o with light whipped cream on top. Snack was an Atkins bar.

Today's exercises consisted of 10-15 minutes of playing fetch with Amber. Took the dog for a 20-minute walk and did two trips up and down the steps.

January 25, 2012

Today is a Wednesday, so I am going through my traditional routine of preparing myself for class. I felt really good at the start of class, because I was able to help classmates work through some problems in our math labs. Since I was at school for so long I really didn't do any type of exercise. However, I did really well on my food intake. I was really surprised at the fact I didn't have that hunger feeling. I am certain that this will be a continuing effect.

For breakfast I had a four-egg cheese omelet. For lunch I had a three-egg cheese omelet and three baked hotdogs. Dinner, like lunch, consisted of three baked hotdogs and a four-egg cheese omelet. I had a snack in class that consisted of an Atkins bar and an almond bar.

January 26, 2012

I had a really good night's sleep, actually had dreams and didn't feel as tired as when I went to bed. Today I ran a few errands with my cousin; it felt good to get out of the house for a little while. Today's exercise will be using the portable exercise bike for at least 30 minutes.

Breakfast was a 4 egg cheese omelet with baked brats. Lunch I had 8 peanut butter crackers. Supper was a rib eye steak with asparagus. Snack was peanut butter crackers with dessert being sugar free jello.

January 27, 2012

After having such a good day the day before, today was bad in comparison. Starting out I had a really hard time sleeping. During the night I over-thought things and ended up depressing myself, which is not a good thing. However I was able to curb the need-to-eat feeling. I was able to finally get some sleep and the day seemed to be better until about 6:00 p.m. I went out with my brother, and unfortunately, he hit a big bump, which caused his car to rip a fuel line. At first we thought he had ruptured the gas tank, but fortunately we were near an auto parts store. At the counter was a woman whom I used to go to school with. She had one of the guys check the car, and that's when we found out it is a ruptured fuel line. Still, one place wants $225 just to drop the gas tank, which may sound like a good deal, but at this point neither he nor I have the money to have it done. Finally got home and things settled down.

For breakfast I had two egg and cheese sandwiches. For lunch I had peanut butter crackers, and for dinner I had baked chicken breast with peas and a salad. For a snack I had peanut butter crackers (noticing a trend here), dessert was sugar free jello with light whipped cream. Did not do exercises today.

January 28, 2012

Today is definitely a new day. While I did go to sleep late, I was able to sleep well. Plus I had a few dreams. One dream in particular stands out. In thinking about the dream I realized that it had to do with the father issues that my therapist and I are working on. Leave it to the subconscious to help with therapy. Talked with my brother, and he received some relatively good news about his car. I finished my part of the team paper today.

Breakfast today was a grilled chicken salad [and] lunch was also a grilled chicken salad; dinner will be a Voila dinner from Birds Eye. I had peanut butter crackers for a snack. And dessert will be sugar-free Jell-o with light whipped cream.

Today's exercise. I did a 20 minute walk with Amber. I actually walked further today and had a little leg pain but no back pain as in previous walks. After the walk Amber and I did four trips up and down the steps which gave me a total exercise time of 25 minutes. I felt good after the walk but felt tired after the steps.

January 29, 2012

Today began rather strangely. I slept okay, but a dream I had confused me. I was looking at pictures that could have been from my past and all of a sudden the picture would turn to ash or delete itself. Started working on my homework. I had a head-ache after this one. Of course I went through my usual ritual of overanalyzing and spazzing out. Then I finally did what I always do and took a break and came back to it. Things started falling into place again. Hmm . . . it seems to me I should apply this method more often, and maybe I wouldn't stress myself out so much.

Breakfast consisted of the leftover Birds Eye Voila, lunch was cheese crackers, and dinner was boneless country ribs with peas. As a snack I had cheese crackers, and dessert was sugar-free Jell-o with the light whipped cream.

January 30, 2012

Like yesterday, today started out a little weird. I woke up ear-lier than usual and felt fine but couldn't go back to sleep. Next thing I know I'm waking up a few hours later. I really have to get a handle on this sleep thing. I started back on my homework again. Got upset at the computer because I couldn't figure out what I was doing wrong in the finance lab. I finally realized what I was doing wrong, and over the next few hours I not only finished my practice problems on which I only missed .75 points, but I aced the real problems. I felt really good after that—had to post on Facebook I kicked the finance lab's arse. LOL. Waiting for the team paper to be completed so I can give it a good going-over; have some ideas that may improve it.

Breakfast this morning was peanut butter crackers; yes, they were for breakfast this time. For lunch I had two chicken cheese soft tacos with picante sauce. Dinner was two skinless chicken thighs with lima beans. Dessert will probably be, you guessed it, sugar-free Jell-o with light whipped cream.

I took the dog for a walk today. We had a good 22-minute walk; went about four houses further than last time and lasted about two minutes longer. My back hurt a little this time but not as bad as other times. My legs felt pretty well afterwards so I may push it a little further next time.

January 31, 2012

I had a little trouble getting to sleep last night, so of course I woke up late. Once I got started I finished up the team paper due Wednesday and e-mailed it to my team members. I have an appointment with my therapist tomorrow, so I am kind of excited about it. I am thinking when I show up at the office tomorrow I will see if I can get weighed so I can see if the steps I have taken have helped me drop some pounds. Keeping my fingers crossed.

Breakfast today was really simple; I had peanut butter crackers. For lunch I also had peanut butter crackers. Then I changed up for dinner. I had two baked pork chops with green beans and Brussels sprouts. For a snack I had cheese crackers and for dessert, need I say it, sugar-free Jell-o with light whipped cream.

Today's exercise will be on the mini stationary bike. I will ride for—up to, if not more than—30 minutes on it.

This young man, who I will refer to as Mick (not his real name) is a delight to work with. He has tremendous insight and works harder to address his issues than most people I have worked with in the past 20 years. He has been taking an active role in making positive changes prior to his surgery, which bodes well for his long-term success as a post-op. As part of his therapy, we have been working on his issues related to his biological father. His parents divorced when he was a young child, and both remarried. He lived with his mother and stepfather. His biological father, whom I will refer to as David (also not his real name), was in and out of his life. David made little effort to have contact with his two sons. David was also critical of Mick's weight and frequently made comments about it. Mick has made repeated attempts to maintain contact with, and to have a relationship with, David.

It often helps to have patients write what I refer to as "therapeutic letters" to a person they have issues with. The purpose is not to send this letter or give it to the person to whom it is directed. Writing this letter is intended to provide the person in therapy the opportunity to state their feelings, uncensored, using whatever intensity of language they feel, using whatever words they feel like using. The purpose is to "own" their true feelings and be able to share them with someone who will not judge or chastise them but will simply hear them and allow them to feel the way they feel. Any "healing" of the relationship can be worked on afterward.

Mick brought the following "therapeutic" letter with him to his session and read it aloud:

> David, I am sure that as you read this letter the first thing that you are asking yourself is why I didn't start the letter with "Dad," "Pop," or some other term of fatherly endearment. To be honest, I do not feel that you deserve that endearment or type of respect. While it is true over the past few years we have worked on developing a relationship, it is not really a father-son type of relationship.
>
> It's time that you know exactly how your actions and inactions have affected me throughout my life. To cope with the stress and doubt of these adult responsibilities, I took comfort in food, which has greatly affected my health and weight. Leave it to you to point out my being overweight at every turn, which only made me feel like crap and caused me to fall further into my emotional eating.
>
> First off—do not think that I blame you for divorcing Mom. I realize that it is a fact of life, and it was the best thing to do for the both of you. However, just because you divorced your wife does not mean that you divorced your kids or the responsibility of helping to raise your kids. When I think of happy childhood memories concerning a male authority in my life, I only have happy memories of Uncle John. You cannot know how much that I needed you in my life as a child so that I could actually be a child. I had to bury so much pain and hurt that it is presently still affecting me. Because you were not around, I had to grow up sooner than I should have and missed out on the joys of being a kid. I was not an adult, but because of what I can only term as "selfish behavior" on the part of the actual adults, I had to take on the responsibilities of one.
>
> Another thing I realized that upsets me is the fact you chose to have a better relationship with your new wife's children than your own. To be perfectly frank, it hurts me and ticks me off

knowing that my father would rather be a dad to another woman's children more than his own. I cannot begin to express how much it would have meant for me if you had been there for my baseball games, my graduation, and other important events in my life.

CHAPTER NINE

Living the Benefits of Weight Loss Surgery

In the medical community the benefits of having weight loss surgery are thought of in terms of physiological improvements. To be sure, there are scores of medical benefits as a result of having weight loss surgery. Post-ops often refer joyfully to "non-scale victories," which include celebrating the day you can cross your legs, flying in an airplane without needing a seatbelt extender, and fitting on rides at the amusement park. Like non-scale victories, the nonmedical benefits derived from losing significant amounts of weight are numerous and cause for celebration. The following contributors describe how they are living both the medical and "other" benefits of the "Bariatric After Life."

"Today is a very special day in my life. It is my fifth Bandiversary. Five years. In one sense, it doesn't seem like it could possibly be that long. In my mind, it could be just last week that I was at my first support group meeting listening to a room full of post-op people talk about their experiences. In another sense, I feel like I've been at this for decades.

I have to be philosophical about my weight loss surgery (WLS) experience because it is a story that is fraught with both triumphs and tribulations. It is not a story of straightforward failure or success. The band, from a medical standpoint, did exactly what I had hoped it would do. It has helped me maintain a perfectly normal size for five years. Within those five years, I have not developed any of the co-morbid conditions that I was seeking to prevent: heart disease, diabetes, high blood pressure, or cancer. The band did its job as an intervention to my morbid obesity and continues to do its job as prevention for potentially inherited co-morbidities.

Because of the band, there are so many things in my life that I
can do now that I couldn't, or wouldn't, do before. The weight loss
has afforded me a tremendous amount of freedom whereas my
sheer bulk used to shackle me and my shame used to bury me.
Before WLS, I could never have imagined riding a horse again,
sitting comfortably in the middle seat of an airplane, climbing a
volcano AND riding a donkey in Greece, getting into a kayak,
power snorkeling in the Caribbean, and riding any rollercoaster
that I wanted to without fear of not fitting. Before WLS, going to
a movie theater, getting on a bus, walking into a room where all
of the chairs had arms, clicking the seatbelt of a car, and finding
a formal gown were all horrifying experiences that I avoided if at
all possible. I did not realize how many excuses I had made in
my life to avoid experiences that would embarrass me due to my
size. My lap band freed me from that.

WLS has given me the opportunity to know some of the
most amazing people on earth. First . . . the team. Our amazing team! These professionals have stuck by me through thick
and thin. There have been times during my five years that I have
been very, very ill. The care and concern shown to me has been
remarkable. I will never forget being so exhausted and frail as
my first lap band was failing and having my bariatric nurse practitioner say to me with such compassion, 'I think we're going to
keep you.' I just needed somebody to make a decision. I was too
sick and clinically depressed to do it for myself. They admitted
me and got me rehydrated. And then, a few months later, our
two bariatric surgeons, together, took me to emergency surgery
after 8:00 p.m. on a Friday night to remove 'George' and give
me 'Tommy' (long story!). All of these men have had a hand
in saving my life many times over during the last five years.
I could never thank them enough. Surely thank yous are not
nearly enough.

I could write for hours about each of the professionals who
have been involved in my journey because they all mean so
much to me. I am blessed to know them all. I am doubly blessed
that they are all so good at what they do.

The other group of incredible people that my lap band brought
me to is this support group. Oh, how I love this group. So many
have come and gone, and so many have sown their seeds into
my life. I have been enriched by the loving, giving, intelligent,
fun, caring, talented co-travelers who have shared time with me

on this path. You have filled my days with joy and laughter in so many ways. And we have shared pain and sorrow equally. You embrace victories with a zest for living that is enough to knock a person off her feet—and you do not shy away from the hurts that sometimes encroach on this journey. No, you shoulder the load and make it lighter than it otherwise would have been. Who could ask for more? I have no doubt that a loving God designed groups to work just this way.

My weight loss opened my eyes to a very ugly side of life: the deeply real, personal, understanding of obesity discrimination. I was mostly unaware how much I had been affected by my obesity until I became a normal-sized person. Gradually, as the weight came off, I began to notice that people treated me differently. I am no longer 'invisible' to the world. People speak to me and make eye contact with me in passing. Gentlemen rush to open doors for me or to carry heavy items for me. Before my weight loss, I rarely had a gentleman rush to do anything for me. I surmise that it is because they did not see me exactly as a 'woman.' I was just a 'fat person' who could carry that package and open that door just fine. To the majority of the world, I was not only invisible; I was mostly genderless.

It was a disgusting realization when I discovered that I was being treated differently as I lost my weight. Waiters and waitresses treat me differently. Sales associates treat me differently. Even those in the academic and professional world treat me differently. Suddenly, I seem to have developed approximately 30 new I.Q. points. My thoughts and ideas are taken much more seriously . . . or at least I don't have to repeat myself as much to have them heard. Most of us know that fat does NOT equal stupid. Too bad most of the rest of the world hasn't discovered that yet.

And then there's my body's relationship with this lap band. It is no secret that I have struggled with finding the balance between my very sensitive body and this tool that I've been given. I have desperately wanted it to work for me. I spent the first several years driving me and the band beyond the limits of what was reasonable to maintain. I thought for sure that I could find the balance and then simply live my life as a normal bandster. I pushed me, I pushed my bariatric nurse practitioner, I pushed my surgeon, and did I mention that I pushed me? I just knew I HAD to get this right. I thought that I was smart enough to figure out a way to be 'perfectly' adjusted so that my body would tolerate the tight times, but that I wouldn't be hungry during the good times.

It was not to be. For some reason beyond my comprehension, my body puffs up with the slightest provocation. And, when I retain fluid, my lap band becomes too restricted—often without warning. This is not a flaw with the band; this is problem with my body's reaction to the band. The band is a static ring, and it doesn't do bad things to me. My body just doesn't want to cooperate with it. It took a long time for me to accept this. It took a long time for me to stop asking the team to make my adjustment SO perfect that I would choke on my own spit the next time I retained fluid.

I had to give up the ideal of perfectionism. I have actually given up on living a normal life with this lap band. It is not defeatist, it is realistic. That is part of the bitter sweetness of this anniversary. All of the marvelous things this weight loss surgery process has given me make the current struggle still worthwhile. It didn't turn out the way I had expected that it would. But there is always a matter of perspective. Perspective is a conscious choice: glass half full or glass half empty. I got the great and wonderful things of WLS. The rest of it is an ongoing story. I'll take all the good stuff that this journey has afforded me, and mingle it with the struggles of a not-perfect solution. By doing so, I will continue to live a life that is lighter because I am unshackled from the ravages of obesity and free from the shame that weighed me down.

Five years. It is a milestone by anyone's definition. As a culture, we celebrate such events in a variety of ways. For me, there will be no particular, overt celebration. This particular milestone shall be marked with a simple glass of water on my counter as I turn in for the evening. The symbolic will become the tangible as I choose to fill my glass much more than half full."

It is no secret to anyone who has been obese that people make horrible judgments and comments to them about their obesity. It's also not uncommon for people to treat a person "differently" as they lose their weight, as the previous contributor noted. I would never dispute that, as I have heard it too many times from too many people who have experienced that very same phenomenon.

I will share with you, however, an incredible insight that one of the members of our WLS therapy group pointed out to another group member one evening when this topic was brought up. Mind you, I have had four different WLS therapy groups over the past few years, and this was the first time another group member made this comment: *"I know what you're talking about,"* she said to the woman who had shared her frustration about the people at work treating her differently since she'd lost weight. *"I experienced the same thing. Then an interesting thing happened. One of my best friends pointed out to me that I also treated people differently since I've lost my weight. I'm more outgoing. I look people in the eye and offer a smile. I used to look at the floor whenever I passed people at work because I didn't want them looking at me or talking to me. I was half afraid they would say something mean to me. So although it's true that people interact with you differently after you have lost the weight, I had to recognize that I also treated others in a different manner than when I was obese.*

I was amazed and so impressed by this woman's feedback. She really caused the others in the group to open their minds to the possibility that she played a role in how people treated her, both before and after she lost weight.

I encourage everyone to take an active role in your own communities and help spread the word about how obese people are discriminated against. Do so in a positive way so that people will listen to you. Join organizations and activities that help others to lose weight and experience the benefits of doing so. Speak at local health fairs about what it was like to be obese and encourage others to be more compassionate about the disease of obesity. And talk to a friend or therapist about the very real hurt and anger you deservedly have about any discrimination you suffered. Then work hard at being part of the progress in lessening the stigmas associated with obesity.

The following story was submitted by a woman who is making the most of her life after weight loss surgery. She actively began the process of seeking improved emotional and spiritual health prior to seeking weight loss surgery. Her narrative emphasizes the importance of implementing balance into life. She works not only to sustain her weight loss, but to actively pursue growth in other arenas of her life as well. What a great message to share!

My Background

"Upon seeing my baby pictures people comment, 'Isn't she cute! Look at those chubby arms and legs.' As a young child, I was the chubby tomboy. I was not fat but not thin either. Most days, I was pounding nails into boards with my grandfather or wearing my pretty, white party dress with a toy gun and holster as I played with my neighbor.

As a teenager, I was a loner. I had to help watch my younger brother and sister after school, so I never did learn how to make friends and was not able to participate in after-school activities like the other children in the neighborhood. I enjoyed reading books, which I still enjoy doing, and it helped me escape from my lonely life, my reality. I did not make friends easily. I put up with some weight-related teasing, but not much.

What I remember most about that time is Mom, and therefore our whole family, being on one diet after another with Weight Watchers being the one she followed the longest. I remember the once-a-week liver, tuna with mustard, plain chicken breast baked until it was like leather, protein, no carbohydrates. I hated those diets. I lived for the times I would visit my grandmother, who had good things like bread, cake, candy, and cookies! While in high school, I wore overalls because I could not afford to purchase pretty dresses, and I could not fit into the kinds of dresses that the popular girls wore. I was too fat. I had very little self-esteem.

While in college, I slimmed down because I had to walk up and down 400-plus stairs each day. By the end of college, I wore size 10 and weighed 125-135 pounds. I looked great and I could walk up a steep hill fast without being short of breath. I would be at the top before others were even halfway up. However, without all that exercise from climbing stairs I quickly put on weight. I love bread and starches just like my grandmother (my dad's mom) and like my mother.

A few years after college I quit smoking. With my love of bread and replacing cigarettes with food, I gained and gained and gained, pound after pound. The more I weighed, the less I liked myself, and the more I retreated into my own exile from life—called solitude. The more I weighed, the more medical problems I developed. The more medical problems [I had] (arthritis, high blood pressure, diabetes, and sleep apnea, to name a few), the more I hated myself. How could anyone like someone as big, fat, and ugly as me? So I was alone most of the time with no close friends.

In 2008, I found three things. I rediscovered the faith of my childhood and rejoined a Bible study group from my church. I found a website called www.flylady.net and in that website, I found someone who was like me but had broken free. I felt certain she could help me find a way to love myself. So I began to FLY (finally love yourself). She introduced me to www.missussmartypants.com (MSP), Leslie, who helped me learn how to dress to look thinner and not sloppy. To be my best and to look my best! She taught me about clothing style and what works with my body type.

I was at my heaviest that spring and summer of 2008, weighing around 236 pounds, and wearing a size 24 or 3X (early that year I stopped weighing myself because I did not want to know how fat I was!). As I learned to love myself and learned what clothes made my body look good, I began to realize that I must do something about my weight. I met Marla (The Flylady) and Leslie (MSP) in person in the fall of 2008 at a Fly Fest Event and was further inspired to address my weight issues. Therefore, I tried again to lose weight on my own. I tried Weight Watchers, South Beach, blood type, and many other diets.

In the fall of 2008, my medical insurance told the employees that in 2009 they would begin covering weight loss surgery. I started to do research on weight loss surgery at that time. Soon other people I know had the surgery and they encouraged me to have it.

My Decision

In spring of 2010, I made the decision, after reading many books on WLS and having many discussions with my friend who had RNY. I realized I could not lose the weight on my own, and I could not afford my monthly medications. I was slowly killing myself with food. I needed assistance, the assistance of RNY gastric bypass. Therefore, I went to the surgeon's orientation and made an appointment with him. My insurance only covered three surgeons in Western Washington for weight loss surgery. The surgeon told me that after surgery I would no longer have diabetes, high blood pressure, or sleep apnea, and that my arthritis would get better. I was elated that I would not have to pay the high medication costs. Therefore, I had my surgery September 10, 2010.

Like my weight loss before surgery, my post-surgery weight loss was very slow. I struggled for every pound I lost and I did not lose fast like others in my support group. My biggest surgery complication was my throat, and it was my biggest trial during the early months of recovery. I have a tiny throat, and they had difficulty getting a tube down my throat during surgery. After surgery, I could not swallow. I had to stay longer in the hospital due to this swallowing problem. I had many tests, and finally, three and a half months later, I had an endoscopy, and the gastroenterology surgeon dilated my throat. I could finally swallow! In the early weeks, I also pulled the muscles and the anchoring stitches in my left side twice. That set my recovery back by a week or two each time. I also have had so many new food intolerances since surgery! I had to stay on pureed foods for an extra month before my pouch would handle soft food. Therefore, recovery was difficult for me. Still, I have lost 77 pounds. I am only 16 pounds away from a normal BMI. It does not really matter if I reach that number on the scale or not. The RNY is the best decision I ever made.

The Result

As my naturopath told me recently 'You are THRIVING!' He told me that my gastric bypass surgery was the best thing I could have done for my health! He also told me that all my nutrient levels were great and that he wished his other patients had levels as good as mine. My doctors say I am unique for a gastric bypass patient. They cannot figure out how my body is absorbing nutrients so well, but they are happy it is. As part of my maintenance program, I attend weight loss surgery support groups, both online (the Gastric Bypass Sparklers at Sparkpeople.com,) and a local support group. I attend weight loss surgery conferences, which inspire me to press on to a healthier future. I continue to work on my food issues.

My Goal

My original goal at the time of surgery was to be healthy, have a BMI in normal range, and be off my medications. I never have been able to get off all of my medications, as promised by my surgeon before surgery. However, all my medical conditions are much better and I feel alive and well. I am thriving! Therefore, a new life goal was necessary. This is my life goal: I will live it anew every day.

My Life Goal is to be active in life, faith, and my Christian community. To fulfill that goal I must be at a healthy weight, actively involved in activities, and exercising more days than not.

Today, I feel better and move better. I exercise regularly and am off some of my medication. My health has improved significantly. I love life and am thriving! So, three cheers for gastric bypass surgery! It is a life-changing weight loss tool."

The next author shares her story of reclaiming health through weight loss surgery. She also sheds light on the importance of addressing all the areas of life and maintaining balance. I love how she notes that stress is inherent in life, regardless of what stage of life we are in. She makes me smile as she speaks about the *"Gotta Do 'Ems"* that I refer to in *Eat It Up!,* and the demands of others, or as she refers to them, the *"I-Need-You-To-Do-Ems!"* She also bravely shares the importance of her faith, keeping that central to balance her in life, and tells how she chooses to give back to others. Another reason I treasure her story is the beautiful love story of 40 years that she and her husband share. I know you'll enjoy that, as well. Finally, I thank this woman for her eloquent praise of my book, *Eat It Up!*

"I am the eighth daughter in a family of eleven siblings. I am only five feet tall, the shortest in the family, too. I grew up being 'southern farm fed' on fried chicken, potatoes, cornbread, peas and butter beans, biscuits and gravy. I remember always feeling fat, and comparing myself to all of my slender sisters. Even though I never weighed over 115 pounds, I always felt that I was fat. With my poor eating habits and lack of consistent exercising, I suppose I was doomed to get fat.

I am by nature high-strung, and very demanding of myself. This character weakness has always been in direct opposition to my knowledge that I was fearfully and wonderfully made. I have staunch faith in God the Father, and His Son, Jesus Christ. It has taken me a lifetime to learn that the high ideals I have for myself cannot be translated to, nor expected of others who are close to me.

I got married at 16 years old, and had my first child when I was 17. My third son was born when I was 20, and my children were my entire life. Like my mother before me, I was devoted to my family, but I never took the time to take care of myself. I lived a stressful life as a Navy wife and mother, in addition to helping care for my aging mother for a number of years.

I started really gaining weight in 1981 after my youngest son stopped nursing. I gained about 10 pounds a year for about eight or nine years. Then I stayed around 200 pounds for a number of years. By the time I was 43 years old, my children were grown and had moved out on their own. My husband became disabled, and I went back to college to finish my teaching degree so that I could replace his loss of income. Of course, these changes brought more stress into my life.

By the time I graduated college in 2004, I weighed 235 pounds. I thought that teaching third-grade students would undoubtedly help me to lose weight, but I never imagined how stressful being a teacher could be. Working 10- and 12-hour days and never feeling that I was caught up was completely more stressful than I could have ever imagined. Then, when you compound that hectic lifestyle with the added stressors that come from the lives of married children and having eight grandchildren of various ages, it is staggering!

My change of mind and heart came in December of 2008. I had gained up to a whopping 269 pounds. I had developed the habit of coming in from school between 5:00 and 8:00 p.m., and going directly to my recliner because I hadn't the energy to do anything more. I would sit there until I went to bed around 11:00

or 12:00 o'clock. I was discouraged, depressed, and lonely! I was taking medication for high blood pressure, depression, and pre-diabetes. I had sleep apnea, and I was a heart attack or stroke just waiting to happen. I would never have considered abusing drugs, smoking, or even drinking alcohol, but I had (and still struggle with) a severe addiction to carbohydrates.

I remember very clearly the evening I sat in my recliner, and earnestly prayed to my faithful, loving Lord, 'Dear God, I am not effective for you like this. I can't do what I would do, or what I want to do for you because I am too fat and too tired. Please help me!' A few short weeks after that prayer, I was watching TV and saw a commercial for the lap band surgery. I talked to my doctor about it, and she referred me to a bariatric surgeon. With the strength that I received from God, through prayer and reading His Word, I began eating a low-carbohydrate diet on January 25, 2009. I went to the weight loss seminar in February 2009, and by the time I had my surgery on April 9, 2009, I had already lost 47 pounds.

I had my procedure in day-surgery on Thursday, April 9, 2009, the day after my 53rd birthday. I returned to work on the following Tuesday. I remained very motivated to lose the excess weight. For 10 months I did not eat more than 30 grams of carbo-hydrates per day. I walked all summer while I was out of school, and got down to a trim size 6. I lost a total of 135 pounds. I am energetic and excitedly go about my life, doing more at school, at home, and at my local church than I ever have before. I even completed one of my personal bucket-list items last summer by completing a motorcycle rider training class and receiving my motorcycle endorsement on my driver's license.

I know that I am still too busy to take adequate care of myself. I really struggle with completing the 'Gotta-Do-'Ems'! All too often someone else at work, church, or in the family has a list for me of their own 'I-Need-You-to-Do-Ems' that seems to trump those things I really need to do for me. I am still reading and re-reading *Eat It Up!* and my Bible, and I am still trusting God to make a way for me to be able to do everything that I need to do every day.

My husband and I serve the Northeast Florida area as commu-nity service chaplains. We visit people who are in the local hos-pitals and hospice units. We reach out to the hurting and lonely people in the community. We do all that we can to encourage and provide assistance to families who are in crisis or destitute due to emergencies. We will be going to the Tampa area to attend the second level of training for this ministry. We are also currently working as bus ministry captains for our church. I am excited to see where God is going to use us next. I want to do all that I can to encourage and strengthen all people while I live.

I believe that Dr. Stapleton also played a part in this ministry with us. When I read Chapter 7 in *Eat It Up!*, about the Enterprise Center, I realized that even though I do not have the financial resources or the time to become the family and marriage counselor that I would like to be, I may be able to realize my desired job through community service. I still have not relinquished the pursuit of a formal career as a counselor, but the words in that book encouraged me not to sit back and wish without working, but rather to go through the doors that God opens for me.

One of my greatest drawbacks from pursuing a degree in counseling is that it would require me to take time away from my husband. We will celebrate our 40th anniversary on June 4, 2012, and I am still as in love with him as I was when I married him at 16. We were apart so much when we were first married, due to his 22-year naval career. These last 20 years have truly been our best! We do almost everything together, and I am thrilled to see how God has helped us to grow in grace as we have placed Him at the center of our home. My husband is my greatest supporter in everything I do. As community service chaplains we are a team that God is using to further the Kingdom work where the hurting people are, outside the walls of the church.

Thank you to Dr. Stapleton for her inspiration and encouragement. After my Bible, *Eat It Up!* has become second only to my lap band itself in helping me maintain my weight loss and my balanced life. I consider it an invaluable tool, and although I have recommended it to many people, I always tell them to read it while they are visiting, but I am sorry I can't loan it out because I need it often. I always tell my sisters, daughters-in-law, nieces, and my friends that they each need their own copy of the book so they can use it daily like a journal."

I swear I did not ask this woman (or anyone else) to say anything nice about me, nor did I pay them to! Since she did, however, I would like to note how this woman has done exactly what I talk about in *Eat It Up!* She has worked on addressing every area in her life and is working toward balance. The entire premise of *Eat It Up!* is about how obesity has negatively affected every area of your life and how recovering from the disease of obesity requires addressing each area and working toward finding a healthy balance in life. Congratulations to this beautiful woman on becoming active in life and making the very best of her recovery from obesity!

Our Families and Our WLS

In Chapter Four, I wrote that obesity is a family disease. When a parent, in particular, is obese, every member of the family is affected in one or more ways. Kids may be afraid for the obese parent, worrying they will fall and get hurt, or frightened the parent will die. Children may be angry because the obese parent cannot play with them due to obesity-related fatigue. Parents may be unable to attend the child's school and extracurricular activities. On that note, in case you are a parent, let me stress to you that kids *do* want you at their sports games, band concerts, scouting activities, and award ceremonies. Every single week I have 40-, 50-, and 60-year-old adults tell me how hurt they were by their parents' failure to attend their activities. If your obesity has prevented you from participating in, and attending your child's activities, even if it was 20 years ago, let them know you are sorry. It will mean a lot to them!

Sometimes kids are embarrassed by, or for, their obese parents. This results in mixed feelings for the child. They want the parent at their activities, but are embarrassed because the parent is obese. They also don't want other kids making fun of their mom or dad. As I mentioned in Chapter Four, children may be resentful about having to do routine things around the house for the obese parent. A child may then lapse into intense guilt for being angry with the parent, who is, after all, ill with a disease.

Spouses may go through many of the same feelings as the children in regard to a partner's obesity. Fear, anger, frustration, guilt, embarrassment. Mixed feelings about the difficulties associated with obesity. Notice I didn't say anything about not *loving* the obese person. That's not the issue. It's just a fact that obesity makes life more difficult. For everyone in the family.

Involve your families in your post-op life! Kids love to be involved in making grocery lists, reading labels at the supermarket, cooking healthy meals and helping their parents in these ways. I can't guarantee they'll be any more excited about the clean-up process, but who knows? Maybe having you around to clean up with, rather than doing it themselves like they had to when you were unable to move around easily, will motivate them to at least help clean up after a meal!

Kids also love to see you getting outdoors and being active. They are proud to have you at their events and proud to show you off as you become healthier. Plan day-trips together and venture out to places you couldn't go to before. Go to the local zoo. Find walking trails in your area. Join local races as a family team. Have your kids help you form a local family group for post-ops and their families, and do group activities.

Let your spouse share your weight loss process and develop a healthy new life together. This is an incredible opportunity to build strong bonds based on mutual goals of improved quality of life and better health for the whole family. Make it a practice to sit down often and talk about your feelings related to the changes in your lives. The more openly you can talk and the more willing you are to try to understand the other's position, the closer you will become.

Recovery, like obesity, is a family affair! Your recovery from obesity will be all the more joyful if your family is an active part of it.

Dealing with Other Issues

Recovering from obesity involves more than changing your eating and exercise behaviors. Recovery is a mindset, an attitude, a determination to live each day doing "the next right thing." It doesn't mean we will always live up to that, but being in recovery is about putting forth the effort to be our best selves in all areas of our life.

Recovering from obesity means:

- working every day to change the negative self-talk you have battered yourself with over the years
- learning and practicing setting healthy boundaries with other people
- learning and practicing saying "no" to your unhealthy wants
- learning and practicing adult thinking and communication skills
- responsibly teaching your family about healthy living behaviors and setting the example for them
- doing the healthy thing even when you don't feel like it
- working on underlying issues that interfere with healthy living
- letting go of people and situations that are unhealthy for you
- giving back to the community
- maintaining an attitude of gratitude

Recovery is a way of life. In order to be able to fully experience the benefits of life in recovery, you need to peel away the layers of the onion and work toward finding your core self. This takes time and self-love and a willingness to work through difficult issues. That doesn't mean you have to work through everything before you can enjoy being in recovery from obesity. Every day that you make healthy eating and exercise choices and put effort into having honest relationships with the people in your life, and effort into loving yourself, you are living in recovery. It just keeps getting better—one day at a time!

The Bariatric Guru has a post on her blog about lessons learned in recovering from obesity . . . this one is not related directly to weight, but to learning to let go of people who are unhealthy in your life.

Some Things Never Change . . .

Last night I learned a lot, about both myself and about how easy it is to let others control your thoughts. But let me go back a bit. When I was an overweight kid and a morbidly obese adult, I learned that people can be cruel. One of my most vivid memories from second grade is of one day where I was leaving school and getting on my bus to go home.

I was running late for some reason, and as I got on the bus, the bus driver (who I will never forget; he was not a nice man) said to me, on the intercom, "Sit down, big mama."

Of course the entire bus got a huge laugh out of it and I just wanted to go crawl under the seat. I had not really let my weight be an issue before that day, and none of the kids had really made a big deal out of it either. But now the idea was planted into their heads, and by an adult. I do not think this man MEANT to give me a label that would stay with me through the end of my school days, but he did.

Once I grew into a morbidly obese adult, I still remembered the sometimes ugly things people would say and I did take them to heart. There was a time where I truly believed that I was an inferior person because of the disease of obesity and that just led me to more emotional eating and to being even more obese. It was a vicious cycle and I was doing terrible things to my health.

Unlike a drug addict or alcoholic, you cannot hide a food addiction. Your body totally "outs" you. It was a tough pill to swallow for sure and my self-esteem always suffered. It was truly not until I met my husband Ben, who loved me dearly at 325 pounds, that I realized my self-worth was not based on what I looked like and that having the body of a supermodel or a bikini model does not make one a good person or a worthy person. I will never forget my wedding day with Ben. The way he looked at me as I walked my 300-pound body up the aisle was something I had never experienced.

This man did not care about my physical being, and for the first time in my life I was with someone who saw ME and not my large body. It was almost overwhelming and I am so blessed to have him in my life. God knew what he was doing when he put us together for sure. As obese people, we can let our self-esteem be so bad that we question those who truly love us.

I can remember when we were dating and myself thinking something HAD to be wrong with this man for him to be interested in me. How sad is that? Instead of feeling thankful to have unconditional love, I thought it was "too good to be true" and tried to find reasons NOT to stay involved because surely I would get hurt. I shudder to think of the life and love I would have missed out on had I let that train of thought take over me completely. Even more powerful to think of, what would my kids have missed out on?

As a society in general, we place so much more emphasis on what others think of us than on what we think of ourselves and that really can get us into trouble. No one should have that power over us, especially a stranger or the media, but it happens, doesn't it? How many times did you think you were just not worthy of something because of your weight problems? How many times did you beat yourself up for not being able to win the battle with diet and exercise alone?

Changing this train of thought only came for me after total acceptance of myself as both a recovering food addict and as a person of value. I think my spiritual life had a lot to do with this recovery. I was blown away by the thought that God didn't love me any differently when I was morbidly obese than he does now. That was a huge revelation and it aided in my acceptance that Ben really could love me with all of that extra weight. Those things are what led me to finally have the courage to seek out a permanent treatment for my obesity in the form of gastric bypass surgery.

It has been a long time since anyone made me feel angry or upset or hurt about my body image. I have gone from being 325 pounds and a size 28 and morbidly obese and unhealthy to a size 12 (I am six feet tall) and being able to do half marathons (yes I take walk breaks and am not ashamed of that, but we will get to THAT point a bit later). I am simply too healthy and happy and comfortable in my own skin to let that happen anymore . . . or so I thought. . . .

This brings us to last night. I had a situation where someone who I thought was a good friend, actually turned out to be very different and I knew it was time to go our separate ways. Do you ever have those people in your life that are just not healthy? The ones who do more harm than good, both personally and professionally and you just know it is time to move on? I do not encounter these situations often, because I do not let that many get in too close and I am very guarded in business. Nonetheless, it happened and I had to break it off. It was one of those unpleasant things that you know is coming and unavoidable, but you do all you can to avoid the situation. Yep that was me last night and I finally had to bite the bullet and just politely bow out gracefully.

I was totally blindsided by the reaction. Words that were used were so hurtful and clearly spoken in anger. I was told things like, "You haven't lost all your weight, so you are a fraud." I was told I was a joke because I did not look like a swimsuit model, etc. I was told that being this size, (and not a size 4 as this person is) made me a terrible role model for weight loss surgery patients. Then a few moments later came the icing on the cake. I was told not to even THINK about including anything about becoming a runner after having weight loss surgery in my next book because I was a fake for walking part of my half marathon. WOW! REALLY? Many of us are familiar with the Jeff Galloway interval running/walking program and know it is a safe and healthy way to run.

I was so hurt!

WAIT! STOP THE PRESSES! Did I just do EXACTLY what this person wanted me to do? Feel hurt? But, the new me doesn't DO THAT! The new and improved me knows that dress size and being able to model a bikini in a magazine does not equal health!! The new and healthier me just left an appointment with my doctor last week where I was praised for my success and the size of my dress never came up. For a split second, I, The Bariatric Guru, the person whose mission in life is to help other weight loss surgery patients, actually looked at my husband and said, "Ben, is she right? Am I really a fat failure and a joke for not looking like her?" He just looked at me dumbfounded. And just that quick, it hit me.

WHAT WAS I DOING? WHAT WAS I LETTING this person do TO ME?

I realized quickly that this feeling of inadequacy was left over from the old me. Then suddenly, I went from that feeling to one of being hurt. Then quickly to one of anger. How dare this person question my health and success and worthiness to work with my bariatric community? I, for one second, contemplated a scathing reply. Then my spiritual side took over, thank God.

I had to realize that people who lash out and attack others are feeling inadequate themselves and just do not know how to deal with their feelings and want to blame others for their bad feelings. My emotions quickly turned to pity for this person. I really did feel pity that someone could be so ugly and hateful and thoughtless. Professionalism aside, would it make me feel any better to lash back? No, not really. Okay, sure, I am human—so yes, maybe for a moment it would feel good. BUT in the long run, I would be no better than this person if I did that so I kept my short reply pretty sterile and included my well wishes and told her I would be praying for her. That was so hard. But I really did ask God to help this person.

The people in my life who share love with me are the ones who really matter. They make me feel loved along with the rest of my extended friends and family and listeners and WLS (weight loss surgery) second family. I have to remember them all when I encounter something like this situation. I am so blessed to be a part of this big, loving, extended family that is the WLS community.

The old me, who didn't feel much love towards myself, would have let this eat me up and I would likely have been very unprofessional and unkind in my reply. I realized last night that even as we recover, it is still easy to let ourselves slip back into the self-doubt and into wondering if we are a success and into comparing our body to someone else's to "measure" our level of success. That is SO UNHEALTHY! We are all different and have different weights and sizes that are right for us and are a good healthy place for us to be. I urge all of my WLS family to really take this to heart and know that you are all wonderful, beautiful people who are on a mission to improve your life and health. No matter where you end up, you must love yourself and not ever let anyone make you feel inadequate again, even for a split second.

Easier said than done as I proved last night, right? We are all in fact human, and yes, just like it happened to the ever-confident Erin Akey last night, it will happen to you. When it does, just remember how far you have come to change and improve your life and to TAKE BACK CONTROL and then you too, like me, will snap right out of it once more.

I would also encourage you, during times when you feel bad or like you are not a success to surround yourself with people who know the truth and know you are a success. There are some great people in this community with excellent blogs and lessons to be had on this very topic. Check them out for positive inspiration.

Besides the love and support of Ben, one thing that really helped me last night going through all of this was to be able to talk to some of my good friends in this community and my best friend who is not part of this community and to hear the reaffirmation that I am of value. I guess we are never truly recovered or immune, are we? But that is okay. That is what makes us REAL. What service would I be doing if I lied and said, "Oh no . . . that person's ugly comments did not bother me."—NONE!

I also took a few minutes and went back and read some of the email and comment cards following last Saturday's Bariatric Breakthrough Challenge, and that helped tremendously. If you are able to touch even one person along this journey and make them feel better about themselves, then you have done a huge service to this community. Never forget that! And never, ever let anyone steal control of your emotions or self-worth! And remember, before you ever get angry and lash out at another, think about how those words can hurt. Ask yourself if it is really worth it. Chances are it is not. Love to you all! (www.bariatric-guru.com)

No wonder she's the Guru! Such great suggestions for choosing recovery. Erin could have drowned in feeling badly about herself after what happened. But she chose *not* to beat herself up. She opted to reach out to people who know and love her and who have her best interests at heart. She took responsibility to get her need for affirmation met rather than to have a pity party and start beating herself up. She set boundaries for herself and recognized that the person she was dealing with was not a true friend. She didn't go get a bag of Doritos to try to forget the problem in front of her. She dealt with it directly. She made a healthy choice to let that relationship go from her life and she chose to reach out to her closest friends for support. THAT is living recovery from obesity.

We can all learn from Erin's example of "letting go" of an unhealthy person in our life. In the same way, we need to look at every area of life and, if necessary, do what they say in the 12-step world: "change playgrounds and playmates." This is all part of setting healthy boundaries, something that may have been difficult to do when you were obese.

I've heard many people say that before they lost weight they sometimes refrained from sharing their opinion if it differed from the crowd, or they held back from setting boundaries with people. They did these things because they wanted people to like or accept them. After they lose weight, they have more self-confidence and aren't willing to put up with some things they used to. When this happens, they are more willing to "change playmates," or quit socializing with certain people who may not have been good for them in the first place. People who take advantage of you, people who don't consider your needs or wants in a relationship, people who engage in behaviors that go against your value system, and people who don't respect your new, healthy lifestyle are "playmates" you may want to let go.

"Playgrounds" you may choose to avoid after having weight loss surgery include buffets, cruises (if you go primarily for the food), office birthday parties, bakeries, and any other places you don't feel "safe" in. You'll have to determine these things for yourself, as every person is different. The point is, in your recovery from obesity, you need to set firm, healthy boundaries for yourself in terms of the people you associate with and the places you frequent.

Thank you, Erin, you Bariatric Guru, for sharing that painful, but fruitful lesson. Erin, along with several others known in the WLS community for helping others, demonstrate another important aspect of living in recovery from obesity: Passing it On, Paying it Forward, Giving It Back . . . call it what you want. It's generous and loving and a win-win, and what the next chapter is all about.

This Will Be Our Day

We will conquer those things that hold us back

Yes, Nothing will hold us back

No, nothing

We are on our way to a new self

A self that will not be held back by this body

No longer bound by its chains

So with my whole heart here I go

Knowing what I'm doing today will put things right

A stronger self
A more able self
A more active self
A more energetic self
A more enduring self

Yes, we will start seeing ourselves as we are meant to be

A more assertive self
A more healthy self
A more courageous self
A more dynamic self
A more powerful self

We will be victorious, because

This is our day

—Andrew Martin, January 14, 2011

CHAPTER TEN

Paying It Forward

If you've ever heard me talk at a workshop or conference, then you will have undoubtedly heard me say these words: "You can't keep it if you don't give it away." I'm not unique in saying this. I can think of many leaders in the WLS community whom I have heard share these same words of wisdom: Yvonne McCarthy (Bariatric Girl), Cari De La Cruz (BariatricAfterLife), Erin Akey (Bariatric Guru), Maryellen Ruggiero (LIPOLady), and many others.

This chapter is about "Giving it away so you can keep it." First, maybe I should explain a little about what this means and where it comes from. To my knowledge, anyway—this is an AA recovery slogan (one of many wonderful recovery slogans). "You can't keep it if you don't give it away" refers to one's own recovery. Recovery meaning, making healthy decisions, one at a time, each and every day. Being in recovery means maintaining a positive attitude and when stinkin' thinkin' rears its ugly head, getting right back on track. Being in recovery means reaching out and asking for help when you need it and counting on others who have been down the same road to steer you on the healthy path. Being in recovery also means sharing with others what you have freely been given by others, including helpful tips for making healthy food choices, ideas for exercise no matter what stage of weight loss you are in, being available to talk to someone when unhealthy foods seem to be "calling" to them, volunteering to help in your local community by heading up a group walk, volunteering time at a clothes closet where people can swap clothing as their sizes change rapidly, and helping out with your bariatric center events.

Fortunately, the WLS community has numerous trailblazers in the "giving it away" category. In this chapter, I would like to highlight a few of them. I know there are wonderful people in every locality who assume leadership positions in the WLS community. Many thanks and sincere hugs to all of you.

I will admit that the people mentioned here are those I know the best from working with them over the past many years. In addition, they have each contributed to this book in some way and have reached out and asked others to share their stories to make this book possible. To these few, and to the *many* who are out there, working diligently every day to make their WLS communities successful, my very heartfelt thanks. You are true heroes.

Let's begin with the story of Antonia Namnath, the founder of the WLSFA. Talk about a trailblazer! If anyone can make things happen, it is this woman! I immediately liked Toni the moment I met her. Her energy is magnetic. She had a vision and set out to accomplish it. In a ridiculously short period of time, the WLSFA has become an enormous success. Toni didn't start the WLSFA for personal success; she started it to help others. And she's doing that in a big way. I have tremendous respect for Toni, not just for her business sense, but for the way she includes her family in her recovery from obesity and in her business. She's a woman to learn some things from. After I read Toni's story, I had even more respect for her. I know you will, too:

"I was born a premature, skin-and-bones daughter to German immigrant parents. I was the third of three children and the last baby for my parents. My father, a chef, baker, and restaurant manager, loved to cook. Feeding his family was a way to express his love for us.

My dad was a Holocaust survivor. He came to America after World War II at the age of 17. He returned to Germany as an Army private to work as an interpreter in Germany. While stationed there he met my mother, a true beauty who had been an Olympic gymnast until an injury ended her athletic career. They married and came back to the U.S., where my father took a job as kitchen manager at Zehnder's Restaurant in Frankenmuth, Michigan. I was born in that small town and I can still eat free at Zehnder's!

I had two older brothers. My parent's first child died before I was born, from an allergic reaction to penicillin. My other brother was the next born, and in many ways, he was a replacement baby for the son they lost. My brother was troubled from day one. He was only 13 months older than I, and I was always the victim of his violent behavior. My parents were in denial, were afraid of him, and were afraid of the mental illness that wracked his mind. I feel sorry for my brother now, but it was hell to live with him. As a child I never knew when my brother would literally lose his mind. I never knew what would set him off, what would make him throw a knife at me, or a rock, a bone, a bike, or a fist. My parents were raised to hide metal illness. In 1960, you did not talk about it. You survived it, and it was all kept in the family, in my family anyway.

Spring forward to 1967. My family took a trip back to Germany to visit with my Mom's family for the summer. They had not immigrated to the U.S. I was already starting to become more 'rounded' than my athletic mother liked. While in Germany, I became very ill. My right ear began to drain liquid as we drove though the Alps. When we came back home to the U.S., my parents were told I needed immediate surgery to remove a tumor that, if left untreated, would kill me within a year. At the time they hid that fact from me, but as children will do, I eavesdropped on my parents' evening conversations when I was supposed to be in bed. I crawled down the hall to glimpse our TV, and one night I heard about just how close to death I had come at the tender age of seven.

It was then I had (what I now know was) my first panic attack. My heart pounded, I became dizzy. I was SURE I WAS GOING TO DIE right then and there! I ran out into the family room and tried to tell my mother, but the words would not come out. I was scared speechless. It was then I stopped talking about myself.

In fact, typing this story for this book is very hard for me. I do not talk about me, and I do not like to focus on me at all! I love to help others, listen to others about their lives. Autobiographies have always been my favorite kind of book. I love to read about others.

After the surgery on my ear, I was left deaf in my right ear. I began having regular panic attacks. I was getting heavier and heavier. My brother was very abusive. My father traveled a lot, and my mother was dealing with her own demons. My mother suffered a very serious fall as a teenager. She had just won a spot on the 1948 German Olympic team. In celebration, my mom and her friends had a slumber party in a hay barn. My mother, always the jokester, climbed up into the loft to make her friends think there was a ghost. She slipped and fell 15 feet into the corner stake of a hay wagon. The post shattered her pelvic bone, and she lived in a hospital clinging to life for over two years on morphine. She survived, but not without a lifelong legacy of pain and annual surgeries to remove cartilage that would build up on her pelvis and block her bowels. In short, my mother suffered— A LOT. And her addiction to pain medication later became an addiction to alcohol. In a word, I became my mother's keeper and my brother's punching bag, and was invisible to my father for many years.

I got bigger and smaller at the same time. My body grew heavy, but my self-worth dwindled until I had such a low self-esteem I was sure nobody would ever love me. I must admit that I can still fall into this mental trap. When I was 13 I had to have reconstructive surgery on my ear because the tumor had left a divot that allowed water to pool, and I was always fighting painful ear infections. On the day I was checked into the hospital, my brother had returned from a Boy Scout camping trip COVERED in poison ivy. His eyes were swollen shut so my parents found themselves with a very sick and miserable son at home and a daughter about to go into major surgery.

The morning of my surgery I was so stricken with panic I was like a deaf mute. I could not look at the nurses and could not hear them. It was as if I was in a Charlie Brown episode. All I heard was 'Wah wahhh wah.' I was spinning; I kept waiting for my mother to come, my father to come. The nurse said I had to take my clothes off. My heart was pounding; I thought my chest would burst. 'Naked, I cannot be naked. I am so ugly, they will see my stretch marks, they will know just how horrible and fat I am' were the thoughts that ran through my head. I somehow put on the gown, but I left my underwear on—against orders. I could not be naked. Where were my parents? I was alone. The nurses even asked me where they were. I knew then that nobody loved me. Nobody. They never came. Wheeled into the OR, strapped to the table with only a sheet that was pulled up to barely cover my breasts. I was terrified. They could not see me naked. No way. No how. I tried to grab the sheet with my mouth to pull it up to hide, to cover my disgusting self. [Those] were my last memories as the anesthesia thankfully put me under.

When I awoke from the haze of anesthesia, I was back in my hospital bed. I saw that my mother was there. I was angry, very angry. I would not look at her. The doctor came in; he and my mother talked, but I tuned them out. They did not exist to me anymore. I looked at the television. I just stared at it and ignored their questions. My mother was yammering about my poor brother who was so swollen he could not open his eyes, how they had to take him to the emergency room. . . . It did not matter. I knew they did not love me. I was done caring about them and myself.

From that day on I began being self-destructive. I started smoking and gaining weight. Food became my one and only friend. It would never abandon me. My brother became more and more violent, and my parents' relationship was falling apart. My father did not travel as much as he had when I was younger, and my mother would not drink when he was home. When he did leave, he left me in hell. My mother would get drunk and embarrass me. My brother would become angry at my mother, and I would have to keep him from hitting my mother. It was horrible. I was miserable, and I had to get out.

My SAVIOR was my older cousin, Jackie. She invited me to come live with her that summer and I RAN out of that house of horrors. I spent three blissful months babysitting for my newly divorced cousin. I was truly in heaven that summer, being away from the crazy life I never spoke of to anyone—ever. If any of my friends or family read this book, they will be shocked at what I endured. One of the hardest days of my life was going back home when school started. Food became my only solace, but I was also starting to like boys. I was now a freshman in high school and the weight had become embarrassing to me.

I starved myself that summer and by the time I went back to school as a sophomore, I was 5'10" and wearing a size 12. Looking at pictures now, I see how pretty I was. At the time I was not so kind to myself.

My family situation was not getting any better, and I stayed away from home as much as possible. I went to school, I worked, and I had a boyfriend. I spent all my time with him. He was older than I was; he was 21, and I was 16. I would drive to his college and stay hidden in his dorm room. Two days after I turned 18, during my senior year of high school, I was emancipated. I signed myself out of school. I packed my things and moved out of my parents' home. I moved out in the middle of the night. I called my parents to give them the news. I no longer lived with them. I moved into my boyfriend's first apartment after graduating from college. I was free. I did not care if it was right or wrong, I was free.

My parents said they would not visit me if I did not get married. I started gaining the weight back. I knew the relationship I was in was not good. My boyfriend was making good money at his job and began a lifelong love affair with beer, lots of beer. I was living with another alcoholic. I started getting panic attacks again. I was not free, not by a long shot. I think the low self-esteem was my worst enemy. I knew I was in a bad situation but did not believe in myself enough to think I deserved anything better. Life moved on, and we got married. I got bigger and bigger.

When I was 21, I was in Los Angeles for a friend's wedding. The phone rang, and it was my uncle, my father's oldest brother. 'How did he find me?' was my first thought. I took the phone to hear his voice utter the words I knew I was destined to hear: 'Your mother died. Your father found her dead in her car.' My father had been out of town. This meant my mother would have been drinking. Her modus operandi was to go to a convenience store and buy a big bottle of vodka. She would park her car and drink the entire bottle until she passed out. On this day in early August it was 103 degrees out. My mother died of suffocation in her sleep. At the funeral we told the world it was a heart attack. It was private family business. I got bigger. The panic attacks were bigger than ever, too.

When I was 24 and my husband was 29, he said he wanted children before he turned 30. He had been an only child with an older father. He wanted to have two kids and be a younger dad.

I did not want to have kids at all, but again, I was so weak, with such a low opinion of myself, I went along with his wishes. I knew it was wrong, I knew I did not love him, but I could not imagine anyone else wanting me. I felt trapped. I was trapped by my own low opinion of myself. Panic attacks drained me. I got bigger. We had two kids. And I can say with the greatest joy in my heart they saved my life. Those two babies gave me a purpose and ultimately led me to the place I am today, but it was a long journey indeed!

I was transformed by motherhood. Having kids did not fix my panic attacks, but those two little people did give me strength. The kids were very close in age; only 18 months between them. After my daughter's birth I weighed 260 pounds. My husband was a merchant mariner; he worked on commercial ships. That meant he was gone for as long as six months at a time. One day while he was away working I had a strange feeling come over me. I had to find something. I did not know what it was, but I had to find it. I started riffling though drawers and cupboards. I cracked open my husband's desk drawer and pulled out a locked briefcase he kept in there. I broke it open, and there it was—a picture of him with another woman. They made a happy looking couple. I was right. I was unlovable. That night my best friend came over to talk me off a cliff. She brought with her a pack of cigarettes (I had not smoked in five years, I quit before having babies)—but that night I became a smoker, a drinker, and a lost soul. I got bigger.

I bought time for myself and the kids. I confronted my husband about the other woman. It is true what they say. Sailors do have a woman in every port! Four years later, when my youngest child started school, I made my move. I went back to work full time; I went on a starvation diet. All I ate was hard candies during the day and one meal for dinner. In six months, I was again a size 12. When my husband came home from his latest trip overseas, I told him I wanted out of the marriage and I asked him to move out. After six months he finally gave me my wish.

After two years I relocated back home to Northern California. I had been working as an events coordinator for a small city in Oregon. Back in California, I needed to make more money to support my children, and I turned to computers. I learned how to program computers, and in the mid-nineties became a very well-paid consultant.

I met my current husband via the computer. At the time, people did not yet have sites to meet on the Internet. He and I were trailblazers! It was so odd at that time. I hid the fact we met via CompuServe. Most people had never even heard of 'chatting' at that time, and it was a very secret world, one that I adored. He and I met on a mental level, not physical. Nothing was based on looks. It was all about our brains. At that time, it was even difficult to share a photo. Computers saved me from myself. They were a tool to make a life that was above and beyond anything I thought I was capable of. I rode the wave of technology, and it landed me in a new life with a new man, and together we took good care of the six children between us. Yes—hard work, lots and lots of hard work was associated with this new life. He and I and the six kids cost a lot! It did not matter—we were making a happy life for all of us. Our way.

It was at this time that my brother died. He was only 34 years old. He had contracted AIDS from drug use and his sad, sad life ended in a hospital bed in Oklahoma with my father by his side. The drugs that would have spared his life did not exist for another three years. My brother's life is a book in itself, so I will just say this: his death from AIDS dug into me like the devil himself. I felt wracked with guilt for not being there when he died, but I could not be with him then. I was not capable. I had a lot of anger for the abuse I suffered at his hands. I now know he was diagnosed at the end of his life as being a sociopath and he suffered from paranoid schizophrenia. I forgive him and myself.

I had a HUGE PHOBIA of doctors—from my childhood fear of death to years of being talked down to by doctors about my weight. It went from dreading to go to the doctor, to fear of doctors, and it resulted in my [not] going to see a physician for 10 years. The longer it was, the worse my fear became. In the end, this phobia caused me to make all the wrong decisions when my father became ill.

I started to regain my weight, and the panic attacks returned. It seems I was very good at making everything and everyone around me happy but had no idea how to take good care of me. I never knew I was worth it. Jim and I lived together, not married, happily ridding this wave. We spent many days in Maui, where we had invested our hard-earned money in condos for our someday retirement. I was gaining weight. I had stopped smoking again, and the weight piled on. Jim and I finally got married.

We had an impromptu surprise wedding in the cabana on the beach in West Maui. It was a week when several dear old friends and even some family were in Maui. We surprised them all.

There is a famous Hawaiian singer named 'IZ,' Israel Kamakawiwo'ole. Most people have heard his version of 'Over the Rainbow,' as it has been in many films. Throughout his life, Kamakawiwo'ole was obese and at one point weighed 757 pounds. At the age of 38, IZ died. We lost a national treasure to the disease of obesity. It was while listening to his music and watching another amazing Maui sunset that my husband saved my life. He spoke to me about IZ and how he believed if he had gastric bypass surgery he would still be with us today. He said that he wanted me to consider weight loss surgery. He asked me to at least research this as an option for myself.

My maternal grandmother in Germany had passed away at 96 years old. My husband and I took my father to Germany for the funeral. We spent a week visiting towns that my father had grown up in as little Franzl. He shared with us his childhood memories and literally skipped across cobblestone streets of his youth. He was 72 at the time. As we prepared to return home my father became ill. We all thought he had a bug, cold, or flu.

On the flight home he got sicker and sicker. When we were getting ready to go to the airport, I asked him if we should stay another day and see a doctor (secretly hoping he would say no) and he said, 'No, as long as I am with you I will be okay.' As we began our flight home, my father was sweating and weak. He was suffering from a heart attack but I did not know the signs. He did not have a pain in his arm or shoulder or chest. I asked him if his heart was okay. He said he had just had a checkup, and the doctor said he did not see any heart issues. I was relieved but still worried.

Our plane from Frankfurt to New York was part of a terrorist bomb scare! The captain came on and told us we were making an emergency landing in England. I looked around the plane, my heart pounding, my sick father by my side. My only thought was, 'I have to see my children one more time.' My husband Jim was trying to reassure both my dad and me. The plane began dumping fuel; it was a fully loaded 747, and they cannot land with a full tank of gasoline. The cabin crew began searching the inside of the plane, opening all the overhead bins one by one. I was spinning with fear. After an hour of dumping fuel, we landed in England, and we were taken off the plane onto the tarmac. My dad was so weak he had to use a wheelchair. In England, I again asked dad if he wanted to see a doctor. He kept insisting he was just ill with a bug and wanted to get home. If I had not been so afraid of all things medical, I know I would have forced him to see a doctor. But my phobia was relieved each time he said no.

After the plane was cleared, we all got back on and flew to New York. This episode added about six hours to an already long 12-hour flight to get to California. In New York, Dad was still sweaty but feeling a bit better and even ate some lunch. We boarded our final plane home to California and arrived at our home at 3:00 o'clock in the morning. I put my father to bed with cold medicine and instructions that in the morning if he was not feeling better we would see a doctor. He never woke up. I never forgave myself. I gained a lot of weight.

I also knew I was on a path to an early death. I was morbidly obese, suffering from Pickwickian syndrome. It meant I needed oxygen at night because the extra weight I carried, mostly in my torso, was too heavy for my lungs to operate properly when lying down. I would wake up exhausted, as if I had never slept. One night I woke up completely deprived of oxygen. I was purple, and when I stood up, I fell down to the floor and felt like I was going to die. Like many nights, I had not worn my oxygen, and my body could not take it. It was the moment I finally knew I needed help. I had to face my fears and get help to save my life.

Jim's words to me about weight loss surgery were screaming in my brain! I took his words to heart and began researching. I found thousands of people's stories on YouTube! I spent months watching videos and learning about all my options. On May 18, 2009, I had gastric bypass surgery, and my life was changed in every way a life could be. It was the best decision of my life, and I will always be grateful to my husband for being brave and talking to me about getting medical treatment for my obesity. I will also be forever grateful to YouTube's 'MassageGoddess,' Ms. Amelia Hall, for inspiring me and teaching me what it really meant to be a weight loss surgery patient. I screwed up my courage, and for the first time in many years went to the doctor and asked for help!

Today, three years later, I am at the healthy weight of 188 pounds. I have stayed at this weight for over two years and for the first time in my 51years on this earth, I feel normal. In my first year as a post-op, I joined about 60 fellow YouTube weight loss surgery patients at a gathering in Las Vegas at a meet-and-greet. It was there I learned how many people are denied weight loss surgery by their insurance companies. It was also there that I met Rosemary and learned about her identical twin sister, Connie, who had been fighting for 10 years to have weight loss surgery. And it was there I had an epiphany, my 'aha' moment. I found out WHY I was put on this earth. It was to start a non-profit organization to help people get weight loss surgery, and the Weight Loss Surgery Foundation was born.

Three months later the WLSFA was incorporated and today we are an official 501(C)3 public charity. Powered by thousands of weight loss surgery patients, medical professionals, and industry partners, we are funding grants for weight loss surgery and reconstructive surgery after massive weight loss! Our inaugural grant recipient was Connie Bailey, and she remains our Ambassador of HOPE! Together our community is gaining a voice, and we are chipping away at the negative bias endured by all suffering from obesity. People often thank me for saving other people's lives. I am grateful for the role I play in that. It helps me to know that I can finally help save lives, face my own phobias, and make good in this world. I am blessed."

Antonia—thank you for sharing so openly the story of your struggle with obesity and your journey to recovery. You have tremendous inner strength. I trust I speak for hundreds and hundreds of people when I say, "thank you" for the gift of the WLSFA. Not only does the organization assist people to have surgery, it provides a network for pre-and post-op WLS patients to connect, to share, and to find strength. And it provides a way for everyone to give back together. From my heart, I thank you for collaborating with me in this book. Together we are giving the people who are walking the walk a chance to tell the real story about being obese and all things associated with being obese so others may feel safe enough to reach out for help.

Yvonne McCarthy. Bariatric Girl. For years I noticed Yvonne at the various WLS conferences (who can miss Yvonne?). I watched with admiration her open demeanor, her gentle and easy manner with every person with whom she spoke, and her sincere, from-the-soul smile. It was after a couple of years of saying hello to one another as we passed, that Yvonne asked me to have coffee with her. I fell in love with her immediately as we sat and chatted comfortably over our coffee. "No wonder everyone loves this woman," was all I could think.

The more I've gotten to know her, the more I see how this woman is love in the flesh. I don't know that I've ever met anyone who has a gentler, more compassionate, nonjudgmental heart than does Yvonne. Nor can I think of anyone I've met in the WLS community who more freely shares her time, her insights, and her encouragement with others. Yvonne has a passion for recovery and understands what that means, so be sure to read her blog and watch her beautiful videos on her website: www.wlssuccess.com. Yvonne shares her story:

"I had been on diets for 30 years and I was still obese. My first diet was in the fourth grade. It wasn't difficult to figure out why diets didn't work because I continued to gain weight and eventually figured out they lowered my metabolism so it became more and more impossible to lose weight. In December of 2000, I was listening to Good Morning America and heard about Carnie Wilson. At that very moment I knew I had finally found the answer. I wasn't sure how I would get weight loss surgery, but I knew I would find a way because I could always do what I put my mind to....well.... except lose the weight. For years I was baffled. Why can't I do this one thing? Because of that, the shame settled in to stay and wouldn't go away: I AM NOT WORTHY! I knew if I could lose the weight that I could probably fake being worthy.

Through a series of miracles, I was approved for gastric bypass (open RNY) and had surgery in March of 2001. Some people asked about the danger, but deep down all I was thinking was, 'Either fix me or take me out.' I could not live another day in this body, wracked with emotional and physical pain. The strangest part of my journey would be not seeing another post-op for three years, which turned out to be a blessing of sorts. Since I hadn't seen anyone who regained, I assumed that I wouldn't. I also BELIEVED I could do it. When I gained a couple of pounds, I took them off because I believed it worked that way. I BELIEVED. I knew I could do it because I really didn't know any better.

I attended my first WLS event in 2004 with approximately 380 other post-ops. It was bariatric Disneyland! At three years out, I was a veteran and people flocked to me and asked me how I kept the weight off. I wasn't special. It was what I believed. It was then that I saw a great need for someone to help others learn how to keep the weight off because there wasn't any aftercare, nor did anyone think we would require any further education after surgery.

By the time I was five years out, a light bulb exploded in my head. We exhibit the exact same traits as anyone with addiction. I admitted to myself I was an addict, and it explained why some of my friends switched to drugs, alcohol, shopping, sex, and/or gambling after having weight loss surgery. Cross addiction soon became an accepted term. Who would tell the new people?? How could I let them walk blindly into this aftermath of problems that needed to be addressed on the psychological level? I wasn't an expert, but I was getting an incredible street credential doctorate. I wasn't going to stop talking until some people listened. For me, it was like watching someone walk down a path without knowing they were about to step off a cliff. I had to tell them about the cliff!

That's when Bariatric Girl was born. The blog, the Facebook page, Twitter, YouTube—All things Bariatric Girl. Even though I am extremely sensitive, I had to put myself out there and try to pay it forward so that others could do the same thing in turn. It is like a ripple in a pond that reaches generations of post-ops, and it must be done until the bariatric field catches up.

After studying the field of addiction, I also learned that 'you can't keep it unless you give it away.' The reason I needed to do this was to help me! If left alone to my own devices for too long, I am right back in my crazy head, and I'm playing those old stinkin' thinkin' tapes. The only way I can begin to quiet them is to pay it forward. At least I now know those tapes for what they are. They are the result of the toxic shame I felt for years because I thought I was a failure and believed it was all my fault. Even staying at goal since surgery has not boosted my self-esteem, because that's not what it's about. Nothing outside of me will make me happy. It's about doing 'esteem-able' things and giving back to my community, and as long as I do that I'll have more good days than bad and realize that the grass is green enough for right now."

—Yvonne McCarthy (open RNY, March 30, 2001)

Thank you, Yvonne. You are one of the *winners* we talk about sticking with! Just thinking of you makes me smile. You'll always be in my heart, and I treasure our recovery bond. Let people love you like you do them!

Carla. Unlike the others being highlighted in this chapter, Carla is more locally known than nationally known. I've never seen anyone in a local community accomplish the things this woman has. She's also talented at getting people to help so she doesn't have to do everything by herself! I hope your WLS community is as fortunate as ours is to have a leader like Carla in it. She initiated and monitors the local online support group, heads up two monthly support groups, started a clothing closet, gave birth to an annual "Bariatric Ball," a celebration for patients and a local fundraiser and obesity awareness event, spoke at the state capitol as a voice of the obese population in support of weight loss surgery, and is involved with the WLSFA.

"I was teased about my weight as a child, but I don't think it was as bad as it could have been. Like most people who are different in some way, I poked fun at myself to control that situation. As a teen, I used to cruise the main drag with my friends. We lived in a small town, so we met people at the local Sonic-type place, so guys would usually meet you while you are sitting in a car. I remember the first time I got out of my car after talking to a guy for quite a while. He was quite upset to see that I wasn't a size 4, and he reacted pretty violently. He was apparently embarrassed that he had been seen trying to get my interest, and even bragged that he had my attention. He shook and bounced my car and shouted ugly things. It was all very embarrassing.

My family used to bribe me with money and vacations to lose weight. 'If you lose 50 pounds, you can go to California.' I was also sent to YMCA camp to thin down.

I don't remember my weight really bothering me unless someone else made a big deal about it. When I wasn't at school, I read books or hung out with friends. I actually had very few friends. I tended to hang on to one person at a time. It was safe that way. I was very much a loner!

I did participate in some extracurricular activities, but only when I felt like I had no choice. Of course I avoided things like softball, running, and anything that required my struggle and my fat to really show. I excluded myself from social activities just by keeping to myself and staying home when I could. I tried to babysit a lot. I used my fat to hide because things were just too hard. I was surrounded by beautiful, popular sisters and eventually, by the highly anticipated baby boy. It was easy to quietly blend in with the background and be the dependable one.

I was not allowed to eat what I wanted at home. There were always comments about my choices. I was singled out in ways. Nothing extreme, just enough to remind me that I needed to think about my food choices more than other people. I was definitely told I needed to eat all of my food because there were children starving in other parts of the world! I was also told about the hard times on the farm during the Great Depression when people didn't have enough to eat. And, of course I was a member of the clean plate club!

I was taught that food was love. Food was the way we dealt with emotions. I was also taught that food preparation is a huge point of pride. I was told I was going to be fat when I grew up and that it would be hard to find a husband.

My parents had a very strong marriage until my mom passed away at the age of 57. I am the third daughter and have one younger brother who passed away this last year. My sisters were very close; I was the tagalong—unless they could escape. My oldest sister was the beautiful skinny model who used her looks, but also worked hard. My second sister was the black sheep with a brain. She was the party girl that experimented with everything. Neither of them had a need to be bothered with me. I was never sure if it was my looks, my weight, my age, or a combination of it all. I just knew I was unwelcome. My little brother was the boy my dad always wanted, and there were very different rules for boys in our home. I made it my mission in life to torture my brother because he was so spoiled and could do nothing wrong. I wasn't on my father's radar very often; when I was, it was because I had done something wrong. When I was very young, he always took each of us girls on a 'date' for our birthdays. He was quite proud (and still tells the story today) that I could eat a huge fried chicken dinner at the lake club.

It's ironic; I used to be alone with my weight issues; now everyone is fat! Yes, that makes me smile! ☺

My brother and second sister have gambling issues. They do not consider it excessive, but I absolutely do.

When I decided to have WLS, I made it my mission to educate myself. This was the biggest thing I had ever done, and it completely scared the crap out of me! I've always thought that knowledge was power, so gaining knowledge was the only way I knew how to deal with such a monumental step in my life and in the lives of my husband and children. I was literally dragging them along with me as I challenged death and fought for my life!

What I found was a complete lack of cohesive information for post-operative survival. The more I learned, the more outraged I became that doctors would do this procedure to a human being and then basically tell them, 'See ya!' My doctor was three hours away from where I lived. However, a small support group had been formed locally. Unfortunately, the group folded under the pressure of too many 'I's'. A handful of us decided that we would just get together occasionally at each other's homes; eventually that grew into a new support group. We based the group on common sense. If an idea didn't pass 'the common sense test,' we challenged it! We helped each other learn and to actually understand what we were learning. I definitely learned the value of actively participating in a true support group and 'paying it forward' through my participation with that group of post-ops. It felt good to be involved in something I believed so strongly in and, as an added bonus, we were making a difference in people's lives!

When I moved to Georgia, I sought out a support group right away. At the support group, I found an amazing doctor who actually believed in educating his patients! He had real conversations with me and seemed to enjoy my common sense challenges. He even changed some of his beliefs and teachings! I ended up helping with that support group and eventually working and volunteering for that doctor. Quite unexpectedly, I began to work and volunteer for his partners, too. Before long, I found myself teaching again, creating programs and planning events. I've even done a little political advocacy! The Georgia chapter of the American College of Surgeons circulated a letter to the editor that I wrote to encourage support of a state health initiative. We offered testimony to the House Health Committee as it considered restoration of coverage for bariatric surgery for the State Employees Health Benefits Plan. How crazy is that?! I guess I'm truly proof that one voice can make a difference when it is joined with others! I've even gotten brave enough to make TV commercials!

You would think volunteering or working to do good things with and for people would be easy. Strangely enough, it's pretty hard! It seems like the more you do, the more that's expected. It's a challenge to go from being invisible to being highly visible. It seems that the brighter your light shines, the harder people work to dim it. It's still a pretty new thing for me, and it's very disheartening! It's easy to get lost in the need and bogged down by the pettiness; I see why people get burnt out. Sadly, I find myself getting to the point where helping is beginning to hurt too much. I think that happens to many of us. Setting boundaries and sticking to them can mean walking away from someone that needs help! That's an extremely hard thing for me to do if I believe I can make a difference. I'm pretty sure that goes back to me being the dependable one in my family. That's a role I hold everywhere I go!"

Carla—thank you for the work that you do in our local community and on the state level. Due to your involvement with the WLSFA, your leadership skills will now be utilized on a national level. You represent the hundreds of local WLS leaders and the work they do to help others throughout the country. Thank you and big hugs to you all.

Maryellen Ruggiero. LIPOLady. I hope I get the opportunity to know Maryellen better. Our paths cross a lot, but usually when we're too busy to sit down and really chat. I have memories of some silly, playful fun a group of us had one afternoon with a blender, a variety of protein drinks, and a video camera! Maryellen knows how to laugh and have fun. And, without a doubt, this woman knows how to build an organization! LIPO may be the largest support group in the country. I can't say for sure, but I can say with certainty that Maryellen has done one heck of a job organizing that group into a dynamic support group that combines education, involvement, and a whole lot of fun into one package! Maryellen is using her gifts and talents in the most worthwhile way: helping others and teaching them to help themselves as well. Seems Maryellen was born to do LIPO:

Paying It Forward

"Sono molto fiera di essere della discendenza italiana e la cultura contiene molte benedizioni. (I am very proud to be of Italian descent and the culture contains many blessings.) We are very proud and extremely passionate people. That passion flavors our behavior in many facets of our life. We laugh quickly and cry with feeling.

I grew up in a predominantly Italian neighborhood, with cousins down the block and across the street. If not by blood, my neighbors were 'family' by tradition. When we celebrated a birth or communion, or mourned the loss of one of our own, we gathered together as a community, and we ate. Every family participated by making a favorite dish in quantities sufficient to guarantee everyone could have at least a second helping. I don't blame my heritage for my struggle with weight issues, but merely point out we develop our eating habits at an early age. Those habits can be related to cultural influences.

I have struggled with my weight as long as I can remember. I began my first diet at approximately 10 years old and have unsuccessfully dieted ever since. Before weight loss surgery, my experience with dieting was terrible; it was the only subject that I failed repeatedly. I had tried numerous diets such as Weight Watchers, Jenny Craig, Nutrisystem, Overeaters Anonymous, along with any crazy fad diet that was suggested to me such as the grapefruit diet, the veggie soup diet, and probably the craziest of all, the frankfurter and vanilla ice cream diet, only to lose a lot of weight quickly but to regain it all back and then some!

Growing up, I was the exception rather than the rule. I was the first of my friends to 'develop.' I hated gym class for the obvious reasons, having to buy my gym clothes in the adult section of the store. As an early 'bloomer,' I celebrated (?) 'womanhood' at 10 years old and struggled with the onslaught of hormonal changes and ensuing depression. My answer to this issue became a food addiction and this was the start of my yo-yo weight history.

Although popular, I felt excluded in most social settings due to my weight; filling the role of 'the fat friend.' In my mid-teens, a comment that I will never forget was made by a family member and sent me into my worst weight gain: 'Maryellen, your belly is bigger than your boobs.' I was well aware of the problem but had no tools to properly respond in order to gain control of the vicious cycle of losing and gaining pounds.

I lost 30 pounds prior to my wedding and had my gown fitted, only to have to rush back to the seamstress to have it let out just before the big day. I was devastated. My answer to this was to resort to my learned habit of consuming my comfort foods. I continued my destructive diet patterns through the years of marriage and raising two daughters.

I went through the motions of participating in scouting, school meetings, and after-school activities; too heavy to immerse myself completely as my heart desired. I still carry the guilt of giving only the token amount of physical support my family deserved.

Through the years, I became one of the biggest supporters of Weight Watchers, dreaming that someday I could make the program work and actually become a Weight Watcher staff member as a model participant. I rejoined Weight Watchers 29 different times, never able to lose my goal weight, maintain it, and begin to realize my dream of 'paying it forward.'

During these years, I watched my mother progress from overweight to morbidly obese and suffer the co-morbidities that accompany this disease. I also saw her lifestyle drastically change, not for the better, as her mobility restrictions began to manifest themselves in everyday life. My father had to assist with daily personal requests like bathing, hooking her bra, and tying her shoes. I heard the progressive demands that were made on family because of her overweight condition. Very few men could or would suffer the continual support my father was required to offer in order to have my mother remain in her home till the day of her passing.

I heard myself becoming my mother; asking family members to 'go get this and that for me' as my weight began to take a toll on my ability to comfortably complete my daily expectations. I refused to allow that to happen to me or my family, and knew that I had to have help in the form of weight loss surgery. I had met a few individuals who had surgery and experienced varying degrees of success. I knew in my heart this was my opportunity to finally gain control of my obesity and have a 'tool' to succeed. I researched the options and chose, with the advice of my surgical team, to have RNY surgery. On July 31, 2006, I had my surgery and was given a second chance at life. My experience and interaction with other bariatric patients have taught me that my story has not been so different from many others.

My self-esteem has increased tremendously since my surgery, and the positive results have allowed me to fulfill several goals and dreams. I now have a Bachelor of Science degree with a concentration in organizational management. I've earned undergraduate certificates in both leadership and supervision and advanced human resources management. I am enrolled in a master's program. My work history includes numerous years in the travel industry as well as several years in higher education at a local college as the associate director. I continue to be active within my community and have been the 'go-to' person on various community projects.

In 2007, one year after my weight loss surgery, I decided to tackle the Obesity Help training to become a support group leader and founded my own group. My support group, LIPO, (Long Island Post-Ops) has enjoyed unparalleled success and currently claims membership of over 1,000 active members from all over the United States and Canada. Recently, at the requests of 'commuting' members, we expanded my LIPO dream by starting a second support group in a neighboring county. With my Leadership Team, we have taken steps to accommodate this growth, by redirecting our visions and creating LIPONation on Facebook.

In 2008, I completed bariatric coach training. As a support group leader/bariatric coach, I am able to help 'pay it forward.'

I get tremendous satisfaction with helping others lose weight, maintain it, and achieve their goals. Weight loss surgery has helped me attain the confidence to be successful at these goals.

In the future, I hope to continue to earn more certifications in both nutrition and fitness. I feel that completing these certifications will not only help me to continue to 'give back to the bariatric population,' but also to continue to help myself live a healthier, longer life, as well as set the example for my children.

In 2007, an astonishing event took place: the bariatric surgery center where I had my surgery, along with my surgeon, announced that they have been jointly named a Bariatric Surgery Center of Excellence by the American Society for Metabolic and Bariatric Surgery. To promote this distinction, they wanted to film a television commercial, and they needed some successful bariatric patients to audition. I was invited to audition for the commercial to represent the 'successful' bariatric surgery patient.

Since my surgery in 2006, I have had numerous 'WOW' moments. However, by far, one of my biggest is when I was chosen to be in my bariatric surgeon's very first television commercial. I have been called MANY things during my lifetime, but a model has NEVER been one of them! I feel humbled and honored by this experience.

One of the most humorous memories was when I was at work at a local private Catholic school. I can remember vividly, walking down the hallway and experiencing almost an orgasmic pleasure passing throughout my body. Trapped in my own little world, while smiling from ear to ear, tears of joy streaming down my face, I was audibly expressing my pleasure when I felt a tap on my shoulder. Turning around I was greeted by a nun in traditional garb with the most shocked look on her face; immediately inviting me into her office. Expressing her concern, with some trepidation, she asked, 'Are you okay, my child?' I sheepishly confessed that for the first time in my memory I was experiencing the true joy of thigh separation! My thighs no longer rub! I continued to celebrate, and Sister thanked God.

I am finally at a point in my life's journey where I consider myself very fortunate to have this second chance at life. My weight loss surgery tool and maintaining this weight have contributed to my current state of happiness.

Since having my surgery, I have achieved goals I never thought were truly possible, such as running a 5K race for charity and modeling in several bariatric fashion shows. I rode on a motor-cycle, have been snow skiing, and danced with my husband and children. I no longer feel obligated to dress in black or dark shades of blue; rather I shop to match my moods and my dreams, choosing colors of happiness and smiles. Today life is more fulfilling than I ever remotely imagined.

I originally started my support group because I felt the need to focus on more post operative issues and not so much to act as a selling agent for the pre-ops; which seemed to be the case in several hospital support group meetings I had attended. I promote my meeting as an additional support group meeting to supplement their doctors' meetings, not in any way, shape or form to replace them. The key to success is support. Commitment, support, passion, and motivation will assist anyone who is willing to try this bariatric journey. This kind of support has enabled me to encounter amazing lifelong friendships, and for this I will be forever grateful.

To all future bariatric candidates or post-ops reading this, I'd like to end this with my favorite quote. The author is a fellow weight loss surgery friend, who says, 'Weight loss surgery is a journey, not a destination (don't get comfortable). It's a road that we must travel daily to succeed.' *L'intervento chiurgico per la perdita del peso è un viaggio, non una destinazione (non mettersi a proprio agio) . . . è una strada che dobbiamo viaggiare giornalmente per avere successo."*

Maryellen—for all you do in the WLS community, I applaud you. You are using who you are to help others. It is clear how much you enjoy what you do. You seem to have boundless energy, as well as innumerable great ideas. Keep putting them into action!

Erin Akey, Bariatric Guru. (www.bariatricguru.com)

"I was very overweight, even as a small child. I was also really tall. I felt like an Amazon kid. All I can say about being an overweight child is that it was absolutely horrible. I was always picked on by kids at school, beginning in first grade. The teasing lasted throughout high school. Both of my parents and brother were normal weight, so they didn't understand. No one on my dad's side of the family was overweight. I had one maternal aunt who was. I didn't feel like I could tell my family about the teasing at school because they just wouldn't understand. And it would have been humiliating.

My mother was always very attractive and never had a weight problem, so I would never talk with her about it. She would regularly exercise while watching Jane Fonda and Richard Simmons tapes. From the time I was 11, she would take me with her to various diet programs.

My dad would always tell me I had a pretty face, but I didn't feel I was ever 'good enough' because of my weight. My parents never said anything mean to me about my weight. Nor did they ever intend to hurt me with anything they said or did to try to help me with my weight. They always had my best interests in mind. They simply didn't know what to do and couldn't understand what it was like being overweight. My parents stayed together until I was grown, but then they divorced. I've maintained relationships with both of them.

I had friends all through school and they were always nice to me. I stayed active, considering I was overweight. In grade school I played basketball. In high school I was in the drama club and was part of the pep squad. I just never got to run for student council or the homecoming court. I couldn't participate in 'the popularity games.' I got great grades all through school and yet, because of my weight, I couldn't shake the feeling that somehow, I just wasn't good enough.

I spent a lot of time at my grandparents' house when I was a child. I loved being there because they were always fun to play with. Our grandparents spent a lot of time with my brother and me. They also attempted to fix everything with food. If one of us had a scraped knee, they fixed it by giving us a treat. If one of us was upset, we got food. Grandma loved to cook and bake. She showed loved and affection through food.

Growing up in our family was like living in the movie, *My Big Fat Greek Wedding*. But we were a Cajun family rather than a Greek one. Everything was shown through food. Love, affection, and acceptance were symbolized through food. If you didn't finish your plate of food, it was definitely an insult to whoever had prepared it. All celebrations were based on food. At parties and any sort of celebration, there were tons of food. My grandmother never just cooked a meal. On Sunday, she would always cook and bake enough food for all of her children to take home to their entire families for at least one meal.

When I graduated from high school I was overweight, but not yet obese. I got married young and was pregnant with my first son at the age of 21. During that pregnancy, I was put on bed rest as I became toxemic. I gained 100 pounds during the pregnancy and never lost all of the weight after the birth of my son. I was married for 11 years and had three children during that time. With each pregnancy I gained additional weight and never lost all that I had gained.

After the marriage ended, I was a single mother for four years. I remarried the most incredibly wonderful man in 2006. He loved me unconditionally, and that was before my WLS. And he loves me unconditionally now, after I have had surgery and lost weight.

I made the decision to have weight loss surgery while doing hurricane relief work in Texas in 2008. I was struggling with my weight, in spite of having been on a number of diet programs and was physically unable to do as much work as I wanted in the volunteer groups. I had known people who had opted to have WLS but I thought it was a cop-out. After struggling while I did the hurricane relief work, I decided I was finished being overweight. I researched the various surgical weight loss methods. I decided I would have it done, so in 2009, after extensive research and understanding that weight loss surgery is far from a cop out, that's exactly what I did, with my supportive husband and my children at my side. I want to stress that without the unending love and complete support of my husband I would not have had the incredible experience through this whole process that I've had.

I had always been active in volunteer work and after WLS I soon became an avid support group member. My husband and I love to cook and began cooking healthy meals and healthy snacks. I began working to obtain nutrition and exercise certifications. We would share our recipes with people at support group. They soon started asking us both for suggestions related to our marriage, how we ate, and our exercise. We had become avid runners and were encouraging others to join us.

I was working full time, which I have always done, but was envious of my husband's job, through which he had the opportunity to touch many people's lives. I wanted a job that was more personally meaningful. In the extensive volunteer work I did in the hurricane relief field, I had a lot of exposure being on the radio.

My husband also had a history working in radio from when he was in high school. Together we decided to take the information we were sharing with our local WLS support groups and share it nationwide. That was the beginning of our radio program, Fit Living. We then began thinking about putting together a boot camp sort of program for post-ops, although I 'didn't like how 'boot camp' sounded. What we developed was the Bariatric Breakthrough Challenge. We are thrilled about being able to positively touch the lives of so many WLS post-ops throughout the country through the Challenge. And this year we have been fortunate enough that I've been able to dedicate my full attention to developing the Challenge and working in the WLS field.

The other way I love being able to give back to the community is through the WLSFA. I have always promoted this incredible organization on the radio show. A portion of all the Bariatric Breakthrough Challenges goes to the WLSFA. The radio show has hosted a fundraiser for the group, as well. I was honored when Antonia asked me to participate on the national board of directors. I currently serve as the Vice President of Childhood Obesity Programs. I am passionate about family involvement in healthy living. We are currently working on some school programs aimed at preventing children from being obese and experiencing painful situations like so many post-ops did as children. Being involved with the recovering community of post-ops, both professionally and in a voluntary capacity, is overwhelmingly fulfilling to me. I can truly say that I feel like I get back more than I give."

Here's what is posted on Erin's Web page:

"Erin Akey has used her bariatric surgery as a tool to not only lose weight, but to maintain a healthy lifestyle and good eating habits, as well as to become a runner. Erin is a Certified Water Fitness Instructor, Certified Fitness Nutrition Coach and a Certified Lifestyle and Weight Management Specialist. It is her passion to help others as they embark on the life-changing journey of bariatric surgery to not only be successful for a year or two, but for life. Whether your goal is to become healthier and to start a regular exercise routine, or to become a bariatric runner, she and her team can help you get there! Unlike many who work with bariatric patients, but have never been through the experience of weight-loss surgery, Erin has been there and seen and experienced the struggles.

Erin is also the host of a weekly radio show on WAVH, FM TALK 106.5 called 'Fit Living.' Our latest project is the Bariatric Breakthrough Challenge conference series. This is a motivating, inspiring, and lively educational program for both pre- and post-operative bariatric patients. It is an educational seminar focusing on conquering the lifestyle challenges and changes following bariatric surgery. The mission of the Bariatric Breakthrough Challenge is to equip pre-op patients with all of the tools necessary to have long-term success after their procedure and also to help post-op patients who might be struggling with regain or other issues that are hindering their long-term success. The goal is for every attendee to leave the event feeling motivated, inspired, and committed to the lifestyle changes that go along with having any type of bariatric surgery."

I'd like to say that these words don't even begin to do justice to Erin Akey. In fact, there aren't any words to adequately describe Erin (and I mean that in the best way, my friend) or the ways this woman (along with her truly awesome husband, Ben) regularly gives back to the bariatric community. She does the radio show, she and Ben literally work with families individually to teach them how to cook healthy meals, she and Ben are active in their children's events, they participate in community runs as a family, the boys help out with the Bariatric Breakthrough Challenge programs, they are involved in local community activities as a family, and Erin is now spearheading a Disney walk and is involving the WLS community (stay tuned to her website and the radio show for details)! Erin has a new book that will soon be released in which she tells her personal story, so watch for that, too.

Personally, Erin, I want to tell you that you have enriched my life in a number of ways. You make me smile (and pound my head on things). You are honest and direct with me, which I very much appreciate. Your generosity is unparalleled. And, of course, we share that new Grandma thing! I look forward to our next collaborative project, which is going to get all the WLS community shaking their groove things! Look out! I'm so grateful our lives have connected. I love you, and I love your family, too.

Cari De La Cruz. Bariatric After Life by Cari (www.bariatricafterlife.com)

If you have ever met Cari, you will never forget her! For starters, there's her physical presence. Jane Russell with flaming red hair, wearing stilettos! Then there's her robust personality. And her contagious laughter. And *then* there are the words that come out of her mouth. I don't mean four-letter-type words. I mean words that you have to look up in the dictionary (even if you have a PhD)! Cari is brilliant, creative, clever, and the funniest person I know. We met at an obesity event in the middle of the vendor hallway, and we've been working together ever since. I am privileged. Hopefully, you've read her blogs. If you haven't, you really must. Cari has a way with words that I admire and envy. Not only will you be entertained by her wit and humor, you will learn so much from her!

I've never met anyone with as much natural ability to learn something, apply it to herself, and then share it with others in such a seamless manner. What I respect most about Cari is her willingness to do whatever work she needs to do to fully experience being in recovery from obesity—exercise, eating, attending individual therapy, and attending workshops to learn about and improve herself. Cari shares her family with the WLS community—her wonderful and supportive husband, "Mexi-Ken," and her spirited daughter, Hannah. Cari even regularly includes Enrique and Eduardo, her elliptical and treadmill in her blogs.

I've had the pleasure of staying with Cari and her family in their home, which they opened up not just to me—but also my two daughters—for a week! Cari lives in Recovery from Obesity more diligently than anyone I've known. The message of this chapter has been based on the recovery slogan, "You can't keep it if you don't give it away." I really had to chuckle when I read Cari's blog entitled, "Can You Keep It?"

Can You Keep It?

It is said that, on his way home from signing the Declaration of Independence, a woman approached Benjamin Franklin and asked, "Mr. Franklin? What have you given us?" To which [he] famously replied, "A Republic. If you can keep it."

What does that have to do with bariatric surgery? Well, if you've spent any time with the average post-op, you're likely to have heard the familiar question, "What if I regain all of my weight?"—which, (if you'll permit me to stretch the point a little,) sounds similar to a conversation a patient might have with a bariatric surgeon:

Patient: "Doctor, what have you given me?"
Doctor: "A healthy body, if you can keep it."

Bariatric surgery happens ONE time, but the after-effects are felt for a LIFEtime. Good or bad, we all must live with the consequences of our decision to treat our obesity with such a radical procedure. Once it's done, it is entirely up to us to use the tool we've been given. Forever.

Unfortunately, forever is a really long time, and statistically speaking, many post-ops will NOT retain their weight loss. Sadly, not only will many regain most of it, they'll regain all of it, and then some.

So, how do we KEEP it, once we achieve it? In other words, once we have that healthy body we've longed for, what must we do to ensure we don't lose it?

I suppose, like the Republic we were given by our founding fathers, we must be vigilant and attentive to the current state of affairs. What's going on with our hearts, bodies and minds? Are we aware of changes? Are we responsive to things that threaten our well-being?

- Basically, if we aren't eating right, are we doing something to fix it?

- If we are depressed, are we seeking help from a doctor, religious advisor or other trusted friend?

- If we are not exercising, are we creating a program to get back on track?

These are the sorts of things that go into maintaining a healthy body. These are the things that will help you "keep" it, once you "have" it.

Maybe it's because we'll be voting next week, or maybe because I'm a sucker for a great quote, but I'm proud of my nation and proud of myself. How about you? Are you willing to throw either one away without a fight?

What are you doing to "keep your OWN Republic?"

—Cari De La Cruz (www.bariatricafterlife.com)

I'm particularly grateful to you, Cari, and want to thank you for being my business partner in our Post Op & A Doc venture. (www.apostopandadoc.com, www.facebook.com/APostOpandADoc). You are so funny and make me laugh so hard that you make me grateful that panty liners were invented! You are ridiculously creative and a brilliant word wizard! I cannot thank you enough for your contributions to most everything I do, from the continuing education program, to the cover of this book, to all of the artistic and computer work for everything we do, to the videos you make to share joy with other post-ops, for your voice of experience as the post-op and complement to my "doc" stuff, and for your priceless involvement and contribution to the Surveying Your Recovery Garden workshops (people, you want to attend one of these; see www.conniestapletonphd.com, for info), and mostly, for your honest, sensible, and sincere friendship. I love you much and look forward to working together in this community with so many awesome WLS people for years to come!

There are so many other wonderful people who contribute regularly to the WLS community. Each one is important to the overall benefit of the community as a whole. I am grateful for getting to know more people in the past year. I respect and admire what people bring in terms of sharing their talents and unique perspectives. We all have something to offer and can each gain something from the others. Thanks to everyone who works toward helping others understand the disease of obesity and puts effort into ending the negative stigma and stereotypes about obesity. Do your part to "Pay It Forward" and "Give it Away" so you can keep it!

CHAPTER ELEVEN

Recovering from Obesity

"My story is pretty simple, really. I've been obese for as long as I can remember. I remember the embarrassment of weigh-in day in school as part of health class in Grade 4. My weight was 140 pounds. The teacher didn't say anything to make me feel embarrassed. I just knew I was the heaviest child in my class, and I was mortified. And yes, like most obese children, I got teased. But for the most part, it wasn't a lot and it wasn't constant. Just occasionally and usually by the persons who were considered the school bullies. That was more in junior high than any other time that I can recall. I had a lot of friends, both male and female and was part of what was considered the 'in' group at school.

I was blessed with family and friends who accepted and loved me even though I was large. I still can't really explain why I turned to food, only to say that I'd always had low self-esteem. Externally, most people saw me as a confident, extroverted person—or so I've been told. But internally, I always doubted myself and seemed always to be searching for external validation of my worth. Food became my tool of choice to fill that void. I yo-yoed through my adult years, sometimes losing with some success but always regaining what was lost and then topping it with a bit more.

As an R.N. who worked full time—walking nonstop during 12-hour shifts three or four days a week, I was able to at least keep the weight gain somewhat in check. I stayed between 210-230 pounds for most of my nursing career. Then I switched to a nursing job that was in a confined space, which required very little movement, and the weight gain started in earnest. Nine years ago I changed jobs again—to a non-bedside job for our healthcare organization—a desk job—and my weight ballooned to a whopping 346 pounds in January 2009. I believe I was heavier than that previously, but had stopped weighing myself for a bit.

In January of 2009, after considering it for several years, I decided to have RNY gastric bypass surgery and did exactly that in July of 2009. I was successful in losing a significant amount of weight post-operatively. I experienced a bit of regain in the past year but am on my way down again. I am back on track and as of this week, I weigh in at 204.5 pounds. YAY for me. I still have about 50-60 pounds that I THINK I want to lose, but that's not a number carved in stone. I don't judge myself by a number any longer, and I believe my body and my mind will tell me when I've reached my destination. And I truly BELIEVE that I will reach that destination. For right now I'm just so grateful to be on the trip.

It is a physical journey—losing weight and regaining one's health (I am no longer hypertensive or pre-diabetic, nor do I require CPAP for sleep apnea). It is also an emotional one, and in this past year I've worked more on the emotion than the weight going down—but that was work I needed to do too. Life, even if I'm not quite done with my weight loss journey, is better— every single aspect of my life is better today—for having lost the weight that I have. So today, I want to share with you a note I posted on Facebook. It exemplifies just how far I've come and illustrates just what having WLS did for me. It's a tool—we still have to do the work—but I'm so, so grateful that tool has given me the ability to reach for my goals and to embrace myself fully, love myself, and return to living life complete within myself.

Here's the note I refer to, entitled: 'Today I Danced Again'
Today I danced for joy. Yep. Had finished watching *Serendipity*. The credits starting rolling, and I don't remember the song, but I was overwhelmed with joy and just got up and danced in my living-room throughout the two songs during the credits.

I've always loved dancing. I have a natural sense of rhythm and I am a good dancer. As a child I'd dance at weddings by myself before the dance would even start because music has always filled my soul with joy. I danced.

Then as the weight started creeping up further and further, not only did my body get heavier, but my heart did also. And dancing was no longer so joyful. It was painful—both physically and emotionally. I couldn't move to the rhythm the way I wanted to. My knees and feet bothered me a lot. I'd get out of breath with even the slowest waltz. And when I lost that ability to dance, to move my body with the joy dancing brings me, a little bit of me died for a while. My soul mourned.

Music had always been something that I immersed myself in. I had hundreds of CDs in every genre. For many years they sat collecting dust. I didn't really connect the dots until recently. But I essentially stopped listening to music for several years when I was at my heaviest. I now believe it was because it was just too painful a reminder of what I could no longer do.

About three weeks ago, on the very day I'd set my course for my RESET, I went to a fundraiser cabaret. It was in support of a very good friend. I was a bit tired, so I thought, 'Well, I'll go for dinner and stay for the first set. Then I'll come home.' That's not what happened. For the first time in many, many years I danced all night. The last time I remember dancing the whole night was at my brother's wedding over 15 years ago! And as I danced at my friend's fundraiser, I didn't care that my body might not be perfect. I just danced.

And today—I danced again—and again I felt comfortable in my body, I felt lithe and limber. But above all else I felt joy.

Today I danced again—just because I could."

—March 4, 2012

WOW! It's joyful to read about how this woman is enjoying being herself and doing things that express who she is. Remember as you go through the process of recovering from weight loss surgery, that YOU are more than a number on a scale, you are more than the number of calories you consumed in a day, you are more than the exercise you did today and the food choices you make. You are a person. You have numerous roles in your life. For many years, you may have defined yourself primarily by your size. STOP. Define yourself by what I refer to as the "essence of who you are." Who are you on the inside? Compassionate? Generous?

Adventurous? Assertive? Reliable? Enthusiastic? WHO ARE YOU? What about you do you like? What about yourself are you proud of? The following blog post reminds us to find things about ourselves that we are proud of. Things that may have nothing to do with weight.

Be Proud of Who You Are

"Thanks to my Yogi Mexican Sweet Chile Tea Bag, I have a bit of wisdom to share with you: BE PROUD OF WHO YOU ARE. Thanks to my teabag, I am reminded that I must acknowledge myself for who I am and not for what I've accomplished.

So often, the tone of my blog (and many other weight loss or bariatric type sites) focuses on successful weight loss and maintenance. In my case, I talk about struggles I've faced, battles I've won, or obstacles that have challenged me. Interestingly, I don't always focus on just being happy with myself.

For no particular reason. I'd probably need weekly therapy sessions to figure out why that is, but in lieu of that, I think I'll just go with it today: I am proud of who I am.

You know, that simple little tea bag fortune might just be the difference between an okay Friday and a great weekend.

I am proud of who I am. Right now. Today.

Am I perfect? Nope. But, I'm okay with that because (as we discussed in my support group meeting last night) no one is perfect, and if they were, it would be really hard to find friends. Heck, no one likes people who THINK they're perfect; Lord knows what we'd do with someone who IS perfect. (Oh yeah, we'd crucify Him—ha ha.)

Anyway, let me get back to my little message of happiness. I think it is important to remember that while we are our own worst enemy, we are also our own best friend. It's just as easy to bash ourselves over the head—for a 'hit or a miss,' on something we ate, or didn't eat, or did, or didn't do—as it is to pat ourselves on the back for just being who we are. It takes no more energy to be positive than it does to be negative, and how hard is it to just accept ourselves for who we are? Okay, okay, I know some of you out there are saying, 'But, wait, if I'm proud of who I am, that will make me complacent and then I won't be able to change the things that are wrong with me!' Not so fast, there—as we ALSO discussed at group last night (fruitful meeting, by the way), sometimes, the most important step we can make in any journey is to acknowledge (or accept) where we are.

I used the example of when I was fat. Before my surgery was even scheduled, I had to admit that I was not just fluffy, plus sized, bonus size, curvy, bodacious, Rubenesque, full figured, large boned, or heavy. Nope, I had to say the words out loud: I AM MORBIDLY OBESE. The interesting thing is, the more I said it, the easier it got to formulate a plan to CHANGE it! Simply giving voice to the thing I feared the most empowered me to overcome it.

So, if acknowledging a negative gave me strength and power, imagine what acknowledging a POSITIVE can do for me?

Saying I am proud of who I am makes me want to go out and pay it forward, do even better things for people, make me the best version of myself I can be. Heck, being proud of who I am made me want to make a list of reasons I'm proud of who I am!

1. I'm proud of myself for being a good woman, wife and mother.

2. I'm proud of myself for being a damn good production director.

3. I'm proud of myself for being willing to go out on a limb with this blog and share my ideas with the world.

4. I'm proud of myself for having an active lifestyle.

5. I'm proud of myself for enjoying my life.

6. I'm proud of myself for finding ways to be frugal when my DH was out of work.

7. I'm proud of myself for being funny.

8. I'm proud of myself for trying (and liking) asparagus and salmon.

9. I'm proud of myself for trying (and not liking) eggplant and crookneck squash.

10. I'm proud of myself for saying 'no' to the bag of low-fat chips in the kitchen.

11. I'm proud of myself for being courageous.

12. I'm proud of myself for saying that I'm proud of myself.

13. I'm proud of myself for being a smart cookie.

14. I'm proud of myself for learning to admit when I'm mistaken.

15. I'm proud of myself for apologizing first.

I'm proud of myself for thriving—even after four surgeries in two years.

1. I'm proud of myself for standing up for my rights.

2. I'm proud of myself for helping others with their bariatric journeys.

3. I'm proud of myself for not being afraid to share my surgery journey with others.

4. I'm proud of myself for not fearing what others will say when they learn that I've had bariatric surgery.

What did your teabag say to you this morning? If you didn't drink any, feel free to use mine: BE PROUD OF WHO YOU ARE."

—Cari De La Cruz (www.bariatricafterlife.com)

Obesity hurts. Recovering from obesity heals—physically, emotionally, and spiritually. You read those words at the end of Chapter One. You also read these: "Near the end of the documentary *Surviving to Thriving*, Rosemary said to Connie, "You're going to get a chance to be the most awesome person. The healthy person that you want to be. And you're going to be able to live the life that you've always wanted. And we're going to live together." She goes on to say, through joyful tears, "We're going be able to walk together. Side by side. We're going to get on a plane together and go somewhere. That's what I want. I want you to experience what I'm experiencing."

"WE NOW WALK SIDE BY SIDE! When Rosemary came to Dallas we went hiking. We went to water aerobics. Then she got on the elliptical."

These were the delighted words shared with me by Connie Bailey, Rosemary's equally beautiful, equally courageous twin sister. *"My weight loss surgery finally took place on March 23, 2011. I'm having my surgiversary this month."* (What awesome timing!) Connie did have weight loss surgery—thanks to Antonia Namnath, the WLSFA, and to Dr. Garth Davis and the surgical team who donated their time and talent.

Connie shared her story:

"I pray to God I continue to do all of the things I do to keep the weight off. My husband tells me, 'As long as you're with me, you won't stop.' He's always been at my side. When I was heavier, I always feared that one day he would say to me, 'It's time for me to go.' It was hard when I was just trying to get out of bed in the morning to believe my husband was going to be with me forever. So now—he's able to enjoy me! He has always been very patient with me.

To date, I've lost over 130 pounds. I'm so mobile now. my husband and I are constantly out and about! There's not one day you can say we're not moving! My bicycle and treadmill—they're getting used! My husband is a huge help getting me up and working out. We go to the gym together. He retired—just this year, so we have a lot of time to spend together.

We've had quite a journey together. He had been out of commission for two years a while back because he was run over by a forklift. He'd been at his previous job for almost seven years when he was laid off. He had to make enough money so we could live and pay the bills, so he started driving a truck. He was at a large home improvement store in Austin, Texas. Everything had been unloaded off the truck. He was standing outside looking at the stars through binoculars when he heard the sound of a vehicle. Before he could move, he was run over, and his ankle was crushed. No one came to his rescue. Not one person asked him if he needed help. He was holding his bleeding ankle and no one bothered to ask if he needed help! The policeman who arrived had to finally ask someone to get something for his ankle. They got him some lousy paper towels to stop the bleeding. I found out about the accident when he called me at 4:00 or 5:00 in the morning. He was in the hospital, and I heard the doctor in the background say, 'We're going to get you ready for surgery now.' Then he had to get off the phone! My cousin drove me to the hospital. It was really something. Fortunately, he's now able to work out. Except for when his ankle was healing, he has worked out every day since the day I met him.

We'll celebrate our twentieth wedding anniversary next month. My husband had two kids when we got together, and I also had two. We raised the kids together, and they all live nearby. We have two grandbabies—a seven-year-old grandson and a nine-year-old granddaughter. We met when I worked at an insurance office. He had moved from L.A. to Dallas looking for work in the computer industry. He was working at the insurance company, but was a temporary hire through a temp agency. He had been working at the office for a year, and I had begun doing bar coding. Every time he came into my office, I became bashful, right from the get-go. It was so funny—I always saw his hind end because he was always bending down to work, fixing something in my office.

Every woman at the office was after him! He had women like you would not believe after him. I felt so privileged that he wanted to take me out. He got two tickets to the movies from his employer for being employee of the month. I grabbed his arm and said, 'Oh. Wouldn't it be fun to go to the movies!' Then I freaked out and walked away. A girl came and told me he wanted to go to the movie with me on Thursday, November 14. That was our first date. In January we were together as a couple. We got married in April of 1994.

He was never overweight. His waist was like a 31 or 32. He was always outgoing. I was 270 pounds when we met. Like I said, there were so many women after him. They'd bring cookies and take him out to lunch and have a special birthday party for him. When the administration at our office found out he liked me, they had to let him go because so many women were bickering because of it. They actually let him go! From there he went to work for a financial company. The people there told him they had actually been looking for him through the temp agency because they wanted to hire him!

My wonderful husband said he always knew he loved me—he especially loved my spirit. He said there was something about me and he knew he wanted to be with me. I eventually got up to 347 pounds during our marriage, which is when I knew I had to do something. I was going to the doctor every three months because I'm diabetic. The doctor tried to get me to have weight loss surgery, but the insurance had a clause in it that disallowed paying for it. The doctor really wanted me to have knee surgery, but they wanted me to have weight loss surgery first. The knee doctor and the diabetes doctor wrote letters, and the insurance company still denied it. I was depressed—I lost hope. I knew one day MAYBE we could afford to pay for it. In the meantime, I went to Weight Watchers but wasn't losing. One week I lost 14 pounds but didn't know how I did it. It was up and down. As many times as I appealed to the insurance companies, it made no difference.

Without my having any knowledge about it, my sister Rosemary had a conversation with Toni Namnath about my situation. I didn't find out about the conversation or about Toni's interest in helping me get my surgery until later. Rosemary didn't want to get my hopes up. I found out in July of 2010.

When I found out that I was actually going to get to have weight loss surgery, I was in tears. I couldn't believe it. I agreed to do the video to help others have the courage to talk about their stories. I panicked, however, about doing the video biography. I over thought it. I was afraid I would have to memorize my lines. I didn't think I could do that. I was nervous, nervous, nervous. I drove to California from Texas in August to film the biography. The drive was such a long one! My legs were in so much pain after sitting for so many hours. I had to carry a big pillow to keep my chest up just to go to bed in the hotel. I don't have to do that anymore.

It was difficult for me to talk about my life. When we made the documentary, I didn't know if I had the words to express what my life was like. I just don't feel like I have the words to express myself sometimes.

For me, some of the worst things about being a kid and being overweight were the rashes I would get. I would bleed. If I could show you how far we had to walk to school you wouldn't believe it. It was probably three miles one way. We had to walk to school because there were no busses where we lived. We wore dresses and skirts. I could never find pants to fit around my stomach. My legs and behind my knees would get such a bad rash. I had horrible eczema behind my knees. When the sun would beam on me as we walked home from school, I would pray to get to the house just as soon as possible. I would immediately take a bath and use corn starch on my rashes. Mom kept it in the fridge. My sister and I still had to make sure the house was always clean, even though we were exhausted from walking home from school and in pain from the rashes. The boys were all caught up in the hippie craze at the time and were not very useful around the house.

Now my life is so different! I love just being active and mobile. I love being with my husband and doing things we never thought we'd do together; like playing actively with our grandchildren. In the past, I couldn't be outside with them because I was too hot. My life was in my room. My kids are very happy for me. One of my daughters was heavy when she was young but not now. My granddaughter is overweight. I don't want her to go through what I went through and what my daughter went through when she was young. I'm so glad both my daughters grew out of it. My granddaughter has cerebral palsy and doesn't like to walk because of her walker and her weight. We are all loving her for the wonderful person she is, just as I was so loved by my husband since the day we met.

I wear pants now! I have learned I will never say never. I always wanted to wear pants and to be able to walk out the door and go to the store. I have that chance now.

Rosemary flies down here to Texas whenever she gets a chance. She tries to stay at least a month whenever she comes. My sister and I are like glue. I know what she does all the time. She calls me and says, 'Do you want to come with me?'"

How's that for a happy ending? What ending will you choose for your story?

About the Author

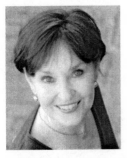

Connie Stapleton, PhD, CADC, CSAT, is a licensed psychologist who has worked in the field of addiction and recovery for the past 20 years, and the author of *Eat It Up! The Complete Mind/Body/Spirit Guide to a Full Life After Weight Loss Surgery*. Dr. Stapleton actively participates with the Obesity Action Coalition, the Weight Loss Surgery Foundation of America and ObesityHelp. Dr. Stapleton is a national and international speaker to audiences of both patients and professionals, speaking at the American Society of Metabolic and Bariatric Surgeons, the World Congress for the International Federation for the Surgery of Obesity and Metabolic Disorders, at the Society for the Advancement of Sexual Health conference and at ObesityHelp conferences nationwide.

Dr. Stapleton's down-to-earth, approachable demeanor attracts a large, diverse audience. She has developed and presents "Understanding the Obese Patient," a continuing education program for health care professionals and "Surveying Your Recovery Garden," an intensive weekend retreat for bariatric patients.

"Your Recovery Conscience" is what Dr. Stapleton playfully tells her clientele to call her. "Recovery is a way of life. The people I see for therapy regularly tell me they hear me 'talking to' them as they go about their recoveries in daily life!" A recovering person herself, Dr. Stapleton shares what she has been given in recovery by "helping others find the joy that unfolds when living free from addictive behaviors." Her motto is "My health. My responsibility. This day. Every day."

Dr. Stapleton's numerous articles appear in magazines including *Nutricula, ObesityHelp and WLS Lifestyles*. She has been a featured expert in *Woman's Day, Pregnancy*, and *New Physician* magazines and has been interviewed on numerous radio and TV shows.

In addition to her rewarding career, Dr. Stapleton enjoys spending time with her husband, her children and their spouses, and her new grandson. Her incredible family "is the result of family recovery from the disease of addiction." She lives in Augusta, GA.

www.conniestapletonphd.com

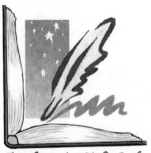

Transformation Media Books

Transformation Media Books is dedicated to publishing innovative works that nourish the body, mind and spirit, written by authors whose ideas and messages make a difference in the world.

Please visit our website:

www.TransformationMediaBooks.com
For more information, the latest titles or to purchase direct

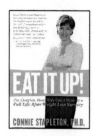

EAT IT UP!
The Complete Mind/Body/Spirit Guide
to a Full Life After Weight Loss Surgery

Connie Stapleton, Ph. D.

ISBN: 978-0-9823850-7-4
Retail List: $15.95 USD

Eat It Up! is the first book incorporating a whole person, mind/body/spirit approach to prevent weight regain in the months and years following weight loss surgery. Written with humor, compassion and a "firm and fair" approach, *Eat It Up!* is a must-have for the millions who are obese or overweight.

> "*Eat It Up!* is a must-have book for surgical weight loss patients. Dr. Stapleton goes beyond the "how to" of maintaining weight loss following surgery to providing skills, wisdom and the support necessary to create a fully healthy and balanced life."
> —John C. Friel, PhD, Licensed Psychologist,
> *New York Times* best-selling author

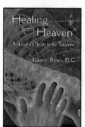

Healing from Heaven
A Healer's Guide to the Universe

Daniel Ryan, D. C.

ISBN: 978-0-9846359-4-8
Retail List: $16.95 USD

> "Daniel is a gifted seeker, healer, and writer. *Healing from Heaven* shares his journey into metaphysical realms and gives voice to the deeply healing power of our own sensitivity and creative awareness."
> Chris Paine, Director
> *Who Killed the Electric Car?*

Spiritual Medium, Daniel Ryan uses his vast experience and extraordinary gift to provide you with the tools to reconnect and sustain your connection with Spirit.

- Unveil your potential as a healer
- Learn to trust your intuition
- Act upon the potential already within you
- See beyond your own belief system
- Open up to inter-dimensional communication and healing
- Tap into your soul's qualities that are yearning to be expressed

Read personal stories of individuals and families connecting with departed loved ones who helped facilitate their healing. *Healing from Heaven* will help you overcome spiritual and energetic blockages to activate and realize authentic freedom, peace of mind and heart, and the love and joy inherent in our nature

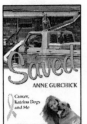

Saved
Cancer, Katrina Dogs and Me

Anne Gurchick

ISBN: 978-0-9852737-2-9
$16.95

Despite her own health challenges, Anne Gurchick follows her passion for animals to Hurricane Katrina devastated New Orleans. Saved through her selfless efforts, Anne finds strength and healing in rescuing stranded dogs. Connect with Anne and her friends on a heartbreaking and heartwarming journey. A true story you won't soon forget.

"If you look up the word hope in the dictionary you might just see Anne Gurchick's picture there. In the middle of her own battle with cancer she reaches out to save some of the most forgotten and battered victims of Hurricane Katrina. Anne's story is cause for celebration and the parallels between her journey to wellness and reaching out to the 'four leggeds' is further proof that we are inextricably connected to our animals and if we choose to listen, the lessons they give us can change our lives."

—John St.Augustine
Radio Host and Author
Every Moment Matters

"Anne's book, *Saved,* is an honest account of the power of purpose and commitment, as an antidote to fear and loss. Anne walks through her deepest fears and discovers hope, humor and unconditional love amidst immense devastation. Allow yourself to be inspired and to enjoy her wonderful journey!"

—Annie Denver, MA
Aspen, CO

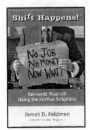

Shift Happens!
Reinvent Yourself Using Innovative Solutions

James D. Feldman

ISBN: 978-0-9846359-4-8
Retail List: $15.95 USD
New eBook available at Amazon, BarnesandNoble.com, and other fine retailers including http://www.smashwords.com/books/view/60296

When Shift Happens you can manage it or let it manage you. Succeeding after shifts in his own life, Feldman illustrates how to stop limiting yourself, retake control and immediately start using change to your advantage. Want to break free of the past, boost your energy, and impact the future? Learn how to apply 3D Thinking to discover innovative solutions in times of high velocity change.

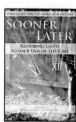

Sooner or Later
  Restoring Sanity to Your End-of-Life Care

Damiano deSano Iocovozzi MSN FNP CNS

ISBN: 978-0-9842258-6-6
Retail List: $12.95 USD

   Sooner or Later offers patient, family and caregivers a safe place to help process turbulent emotions during the diagnosis phase of a serious or terminal illness and remain sane, rational and in control.
   Sooner or Later provides the information and tools to empower patients and their families to seek the appropriate level of care, take control and make good decisions to maintain the best quality of life.

   "*Sooner or Later* is a rare treasure. This book shines with compassion, wisdom, humor, and truth. I believe it should be must reading for everyone. Really!"

—Christiane Northrup, MD, ob/gyn physician
and author of the *New York Times* bestsellers:
Women's Bodies, Women's Wisdom and *The Wisdom of Menopause*

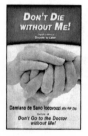

Don't Die without Me! is the eBook version of *Sooner or Later*

New eBook available at Amazon, BarnesandNoble.com, and other fine retailers including http://www.smashwords.com/books/view/105018

   Don't Die Without Me! provides the pertinent questions to ask medical specialists written in a way the reader and provider understand.

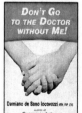

Don't Go to the Doctor without Me!
Damiano deSano Iocovozzi MSN FNP CNS

New eBook available at Amazon, BarnesandNoble.com, and other fine retailers including http://www.smashwords.com/books/view/95147

   Don't Go to the Doctor without Me! is your personal road map through the health care maze from wellness exams to chronic care management, teaching you how to be your own health care advocate. Uninsured or under insured, this book includes important tips on how to get low cost or free services while still receiving the best possible care. All the questions patients should ask.

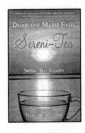

Sereni-Tea
 Sipping Self Success

Dharlene Marie Fahl

ISBN: 978-0-9844600-3-8
Retail List Prices: $15.95 USD,
$17.00 CAD, £ 12.95 GBP

Certified tea specialist, Dharlene Marie Fahl, guides you on an inner journey of self-discovery through the simple practice of sipping tea. Quiet your mind, open your heart and nurture your being as you drink in the peace of self success. Anywhere, anytime, your cup of Sereni-Tea awaits you.

"*Sereni-Tea* is not a typical book about tea. Yes, it contains all the necessary information to help both novices and experts alike to better appreciate this near-miraculous beverage, but then it uses tea as a means for discovering who we are and what we could become . . ."
—Joe Simrany, President, Tea Association of the USA

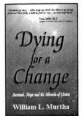

Dying for a Change

William L. Murtha

ISBN: 978-0-9823850-8-1
Retail List: $19.95 USD

Dying for a Change is the gripping, true account of William L. Murtha's fight to survive hypothermia in the freezing waters off the coast of Britain. At a crucial time when his life was rapidly spiraling out of control, William was swept out to sea by a twenty-foot freak wave. Drowning, losing consciousness and convinced that this was the end, he relived many pivotal moments from his past and experienced a life-changing conversation with a Higher Presence.

William's compelling message inspires readers to come face-to-face with their own deepest fears and challenges perceptions about God, life, death and miracles.

"An amazing story! . . . takes away any doubt that there is an energy force out there ready to help us find our way . . . we need only listen."
—Susan Jeffers, Ph.D, Author, *Feel the Fear and Do It Anyway*®

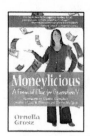

Moneylicious
  A Financial Clue for Generation Y

Ornella Grosz

ISBN: 978-0-9845751-1-4
Retail List: $12.95 USD

Spend and invest your hard-earned dollars in an effective way! *Moneylicious* is an easy-to-understand guide for Gen Y and everyone needing to understand how money and personal finance work. Twenty-something Ornella Grosz will help you recover, or better yet avoid, the slippery slope of debt!

Moneylicious: A Financial Clue for Generation Y explains the basis of investing, banking, purchasing a first home, the importance of spending with a touch of humor (yes, you can buy that $100 pair of jeans). And much more!

"For Gen Y . . . written by Gen Y . . . *Moneylicious* provides a great financial roadmap. Ornella's willingness to share her own stories not only engages the reader but creates a learning environment where the basics of money and investing are not only explained . . . but shared in a way that is entertaining as well as experiential. This book should be required reading for all young people in high school and college. Armed with the knowledge that Ornella shares, the readers will be prepared to not only survive . . . but to thrive in the financial world they face."

Sharon Lechter, Founder and CEO of Pay Your Family First,
member of the first President's Advisory Council
on Financial Literacy, the AICPA Financial Literacy
Commission and co-author of the National Bestseller
Think and Grow Rich—Three Feet From Gold

The Key of Life
  A Metaphysical Investigation

Randolph J. Rogers

ISBN: 978-0-9823850-9-8
Retail List: $18.95 USD

Newsman Randy Rogers takes you along on his riveting journey investigating past lives, present events and reincarnation. Randy proves that "ordinary" people can experience the extraordinary when they open themselves to the possibilities.

The Key of Life is a true story about who we are, why we are here and how we are all connected.

". . . a consciousness-raising self-help detective story . . ."

—Peter Michalos, Author of *Psyche, a Novel of the Young Freud*

". . . a very personal and life changing experience . . . We emerge from it . . . enlightened, inspired."

—Maria Shriver, First Lady of California, Author

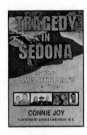

Tragedy in Sedona
   My Life in James Arthur Ray's Inner Circle

Connie Joy

ISBN: 978-0-9845751-6-9
Retail List: $18.95 USD

Follow Connie Joy inside the seminars and once-in-a-lifetime trips to Egypt and Peru for an up close look at the transformative work of a charismatic teacher—and the underlying danger of mixing up the message with the messenger!

Connie and her husband attended 27 events over three years presented by James Arthur Ray, "Rock Star of Personal Transformation." In 2007, Connie participated in Ray's sweat lodge, a Native American ceremonial sauna meant to be a place of spiritual renewal and mental and physical healing. In reality it was just a test of human endurance for Connie and the other participants. Her prediction that someone could be seriously hurt came true in October 2009 when three people died and 18 participants were injured during a sweat lodge run by James Arthur Ray and his staff.

After injuries at his previous events, why didn't Ray get the message he was literally playing with fire?

After a four month trial, Ray was convicted of three counts of negligent homicide and began serving two years in prison in November, 2011 on each count concurrently. He also is facing a wrongful death suit for the suicide of Colleen Conaway at one of his seminars ten weeks prior to the sweat lodge deaths.

"James Ray's debut in the film, *The Secret,* thrust him into the spotlight . . . appearances on *Oprah* and *Larry King Live* . . . *Tragedy in Sedona* is a behind the scenes look at the rise and fall of the James Ray Empire, through the eyes of an ultimately disenchanted follower.

Connie Joy takes you on her personal and authentic journey—from being a devoted member of James' inner circle and Dream Team to . . . trying to warn others."

—From the Foreword by forensic
psychiatrist Dr. Carole Lieberman

CPSIA information can be obtained at www.ICGtesting.com
Printed in the USA
LVOW06s0648230713

343963LV00002B/109/P